Non-Mendelian Genetics in Humans

OXFORD MONOGRAPHS ON MEDICAL GENETICS

OXFORD MONOGRAPHS ON MEDICAL GENETICS NO. 35

Non-Mendelian Genetics
in Humans

HARRY OSTRER, MD
Human Genetics Program
Department of Pediatrics
New York University Medical Center

New York   Oxford
OXFORD UNIVERSITY PRESS
1998

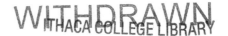

Oxford University Press

Oxford   New York
Athens   Auckland   Bangkok   Bogota   Bombay
Buenos Aires   Calcutta   Cape Town   Dar es Salaam
Delhi   Florence   Hong Kong   Istanbul   Karachi
Kuala Lumpur   Madras   Madrid   Melbourne
Mexico City   Nairobi   Paris   Singapore
Taipei   Tokyo   Toronto   Warsaw

and associated companies in
Berlin   Ibadan

Copyright © 1998 by Oxford University Press

Published by Oxford University Press, Inc.
198 Madison Avenue, New York, New York 10016

Oxford is a registered trademark of Oxford University Press

Library of Congress Cataloging-in-Publication Data
Ostrer, Harry.
Non-Mendelian Genetics in Humans
Harry Ostrer.   p.   cm.
Includes bibliographical references and index.
ISBN 0-19-506877-7
1. Human genetics.   2. Medical genetics.   I. Title.
[DNLM: 1. Genetics, Medical.   2. Genetics, Biochemical.
3. Mutation.   4. Hereditary Diseases—genetics.   QZ 50 O85m 1998]
QH431.O796   1998
599.93′5—dc21
DNLM/DLC
for Library of Congress   97–20620

9 8 7 6 5 4 3 2 1

Printed in the United States of America
on acid-free paper

For my parents,
Jack and Gloria

Preface

This is a book about the mechanisms of human genetics. It was written because over the course of the past several decades, mechanisms have been discovered that have provided new insights into how genes affect disease and development. These processes may occur in somatic or germ cells and may affect either the nuclear or the mitochondrial genomes.

My work on the unequal contribution of the maternal and paternal genomes to human development caused me to think more about one of those mechanisms, genomic imprinting, and subsequently to think more critically about the other mechanisms. In 1988, I was a faculty member at the University of Florida College of Medicine. At that time, I assisted my colleagues, Charles Williams and Eduardo Cantu, on a study of Angelman syndrome, an unusual condition associated with profound mental retardation, uncontrolled bursts of laughter, and marionette-type movements. They demonstrated that a significant proportion of patients had deletions of the long arm of chromosome 15. We were aware of work by Merlin Butler and others indicating that a comparable deletion was observed in individuals with Prader-Willi syndrome and that the origin of this mutation was always paternal. By contrast, Eduardo and Charlie demonstrated that the origin of the mutation in Angelman syndrome was always maternal. Comparable observations were made around that time by Joan Knoll and Marc Lalande and by Ellen Magenis. We postulated that in these cases Angelman syndrome was the result of deleting the maternal allele of a paternally imprinted (inactive) gene and that Prader-Willi syndrome was the result of deleting the paternal allele of a maternally imprinted gene.

These observations concerning novel genetic mechanisms were not isolated. During the late 1980s and early 1990s, work on a variety of other disorders that did not demonstrate traditional Mendelian inheritance converged. My Florida colleagues Tal Thomas and Jaime Frias showed that chromosomal mosaicism could account for developmental disorders with regions of altered pigmentation that followed the lines of Blaschko. Gonadal mosaicism was demonstrated in the seemingly noncarrier parents of children with the severe, dominant, infantile form of osteogenesis imperfecta and with Duchenne muscular dystrophy. Mutations in the mitochondrial genome explained the maternal transmission of Leber hereditary optic neuropathy. Indeed, non-Mendelian mechanisms were being identified that could explain the genetic basis for a host of disorders.

About that time, Jeffrey House, an editor from Oxford University Press, visited Gainesville looking for new ideas for books. He thought that a book about DNA diagnostics, another interest of mine, would be timely. Others shared his thought and have published some excellent books about the subject. I told him that I thought that a book about non-Mendelian genetic processes, highlighting examples from human diseases, would also be timely. He consulted his advisors for the Oxford monograph series on medical genetics, who concurred. Hence, this book was launched.

Knowledge about these mechanisms has continued to emerge at a rapid rate. During the last five years, I have felt the ground shift several times. This has led to rewriting new chapters that were not part of the original outline and to rewriting chapters. For example, processes that are associated with accelerated rates of mutation in germ and somatic cells had not been identified in humans when the book was started.

This book has ten chapters. Chapter 1 is a review of Mendelian genetics. The chapter emphasizes that, as a model for explaining human development and disease, Mendelian genetics was always problematical. Transmission ratios frequently deviate from those predicted by Mendel's laws. Because a phenotype can be genetic, yet not show Mendelian transmission, the tools that are used to decide whether a trait is genetic are discussed. Chapter 2 reviews the molecules on which genetic processes operate. The discussion includes the genes, their molecular superstructure (the chromosomes) and their products (RNA and proteins). The mechanisms by which physical alterations occur and how these alterations change phenotypes are discussed. Chapters 1 and 2 developed a conceptual and operational framework; chapter 3 is a review of the specific ways in which deviations occur from the Mendelian model. This includes a systematic discussion of the concepts of variable penetrance and expressivity, including some of the ways in which these exceptions can be explained without revoking the Mendelian paradigm. The first three chapters lay the foundation for chapters 4 to 9.

Chapter 4 a reviews the mechanisms of normal and abnormal chromosomal segregation. These processes occur in germ and somatic cells. The time at which they occur during development determines the number of cells that have a given chromosomal constitution and thus the phenotype of the host. Chapter 5 reviews how sex chromosomes differ from autosomes in their transmission and expression and in their associated phenotypes. Most notable among these are sex-linked transmission and sex chromosome inactivation. Chapter 6 is a review of the genetics of mitochondria. This includes discussion of the organization and transmission of mitochondrial genomes and the phenotypes that have been associated with mutant genomes. Chapter 7 provides the evidence for genomic imprinting. This process has a parent-of-origin effect for inactivating gene expression in somatic cells. Aberrant transmission of imprinted genes can account not only for Prader-Willi and Angelman syndromes but for other conditions as well. Chapter 8 reviews the processes that cause accelerated rates of mutation. First, the evidence is provided for anticipation, a process whereby a condition can seemingly get worse or have an earlier age of onset in subsequent generations. A germline mechanism of mutation, expansion in the number of trinucleotide repeats, can account for this phenomenon; however, this is only one of several mechanisms that contribute to accelerated rates of mutation. One mechanism that accelerates the rate of mutation in somatic cells introduces exogenous genetic material. Chapter 9 is a review of this topic and includes discussion of the genetic features of some of the more common human viruses.

Chapter 10 explores how all these mechanisms affect penetrance and expressivity—how they limit biological determinism and thus our ability to predict genotype based on phenotype. Chapter 10 mentions other genetic phenomena whose genetic basis is unknown and postulates the existence of other, as yet unidentified, genetic processes. I hope to suggest that although genes may operate in a rigidly deterministic fashion, there may be limits to this determinism.

Who should read this book? The book was written for people, like me, who have sought to integrate these many emerging ideas in human genetics. The reader could be a student, a geneticist, a science writer, or an intellectually curious person who is seeking a systematic discussion in a single book. I have assumed that the reader has some familiarity with the field of human genetics. Those who do not might start off with one of the many excellent primers on this subject, such as Thompson, Willard, and McInnes' *Principles of Medical Genetics,* Collins and Gelherter's *Medical Genetics,* McKusick's *Mendelian Inheritance in Man,* Emery and Rimoin's *Principles and Practice of Medical Genetics,* Vogel and Motulsky's *Human Genetics,* or Weatherall's *New Genetics and Clinical Practice.*

In writing the book, I have tried to confine myself to the facts as revealed by the scientific literature. Despite the novelty of some of these concepts, tools have been developed for rigorously testing their occurrence and their effects. For example, some of the early literature lumped together a variety of conditions that showed a parental origin effect as having been subject to genomic imprinting effects. This has resulted in considerable confusion. Unless there are compelling arguments for doing so, I have shied away from presenting biological reasons for why these processes originated and why they have been maintained. I find teleologic arguments for why genomic imprinting occurred, such as, "Genomic imprinting represents a tug of war between paternal and maternal genomes," to be premature. Nonetheless, the effect of non-Mendelian processes that require a maternal and a paternal genetic contribution, such as genomic imprinting and sex chromosome transmission, has been to lock in sexual reproduction and Mendelian transmission as we know them.

Although this is a single-author book, most of the ideas originated with authors whose work is cited and referenced. In writing this book, I have benefited from conversations with friends and colleagues who helped me to understand specific biological phenomena or to correct flaws in my understanding. I thank them: Thomas Caskey, Sharat Chandra, Daniel Driscoll, Karl Drlica, Peter Gregersen, Judith Hall, Fielding Hejtmancik, Rochelle Hirschhorn, Lillian Hsu,

Victor McKusick, Barbara Migeon, Arno Motulsky, Robert Nicholls, Carole Oddoux, Jennifer Puck, Elsa Reich, Jerome Rotter, Carmen Sapienza, Parker Small, Benjamin Tycko, Douglas Wallace, Stephen Warren, and Huntington Willard. The comments of two anonymous reviewers were critical in helping me refine my point of view. Fielding Hejtmancik's comments especially helped in the final revision. Wade Parks, my chairman at New York University Medical Center, has frequently challenged me concerning the biological significance of most of these processes. My secretary, Linda Gentry, has been a very willing collaborator. She has edited the manuscript countless times and drew the figures that accompany the text. My family, including my wife, Elizabeth Marks, my mother, Gloria Ostrer, and my in-laws, Joan and Paul Marks, have all provided support and encouragement during this five-year sojourn.

I benefited most from the counsel of my colleague and teacher, Barton Childs. I met Barton when I was a junior medical student. My public health project was to establish a screening program for Tay-Sachs carriers in the Riverdale section of the Bronx, and Barton was one of my advisors. Subsequently, he was instrumental in helping me choose The Johns Hopkins Hospital as the place for my residency in pediatrics. During my residency, I enjoyed discussing human genetics with Barton both informally and as a consequence of reading papers together.

After a hiatus of 16 years, I had the opportunity to show him what I have learned. Barton has read every word of this manuscript. In the process, he has helped me recognize that exceptions to Mendelism have always been a feature of human genetics and thus to develop the concept as the central theme of this book. He has been an exacting editor. If this book is able to reach its readers, it is due in no small part to Barton's mentorship.

New York   H. O.
August, 1997

Contents

Non-Mendelian Genetics in Humans

Introduction

During the summer of 1995, I saw a baby in consultation for evaluation of asymmetry. At birth, his mother suspected that something was wrong because one side of his body was larger than the other. Careful questioning revealed that his blood sugar had been low in the newborn period. His physical examination revealed that he had a large tongue and the ear creases that are characteristic of Beckwith-Wiedeman syndrome (BWS). As a result of this diagnosis, we started a program of ultrasound screening for abdominal masses. At three months of age, a tumor was discovered in his right adrenal gland, which fortunately proved to be a benign adenoma when it was removed.

I first learned about BWS when I was a junior in medical school. The idea that congenital asymmetry (or hemihypertrophy) could be associated with childhood tumors was one of the dogmas that was transmitted during my pediatric clerkship in medical school. Clearly, this dogma had an empirical basis, but the genetic mechanisms became apparent only recently.

At least three genetic processes were operating together to produce my patient's phenotype. First, he had uniparental disomy (UPD) for chromosome 11—that is, two copies of his father's chromosome 11 and no copy of his mother's. This UPD was confined to the side of his body that had the hemihypertrophy. As the result, he had overexpression of the IGF2 gene, one of the major growth factors. The IGF2 gene is imprinted so that ordinarily only the paternal copy of the gene is expressed. The physical basis for this overexpression in my patient was the presence of two active IGF2 genes. The UPD, likewise, led to the underexpression of a paternally imprinted gene that acts as a tumor suppressor. Inactivity of this tumor suppressor was the first in a multistep pathway that led to tumor development.

In addition to uniparental disomy and genomic imprinting, a third genetic process, somatic mosaicism, was operating. (Only some of the cells in his body had the UPD.) Based on this observation, one might predict that his other adrenal gland is not at risk for developing tumors. We have not biopsied that gland to determine whether UPD is present. In any case, we are not sufficiently confident of our knowledge of the biology of BWS to refrain from performing sonographic screening.

The clinic is the medical geneticist's laboratory for observing genetic mechanisms at work. This patient and many others like him with unusual genetic conditions have been instrumental in identifying new genetic processes in humans and their roles in human development and disease. Frequently, when I walk my children to school, I see my patient in a stroller with his mother and his older sister, who is also on her way to school. His sister is well and does not face his risk for developing tumors, just as the genetics would predict.

1

Mendelian Inheritance in Humans

After having been overlooked for 35 years, Gregor Mendel's laws of genetic transmission were rediscovered in 1900.[1] Mendel had based his work on breeding experiments in peas and flowering plants, but the laws were found to be applicable to other organisms as well.[2–4] With their rediscovery, Mendel's laws provided the framework upon which all subsequent work in human genetics has been based.[5–8]

Mendel's first law is referred to as the independent assortment of alleles. (Alleles are the two different copies of a gene.) Alleles may be dominant or recessive in their influence on the development of characteristics. (Genetic characteristics are commonly referred to as "phenotypes.") If an allele is dominant, one copy is sufficient to produce the phenotype—that is, to encode it. If it is recessive, two copies are required.

Mendel stated the law this way (page 326), "If A be taken as denoting one of the two constant characters, for instance the dominant, a, the recessive, and Aa the hybrid form in which both are conjoined, the expression $A + 2Aa + a$ shows the terms in the series for the progeny of the hybrids of two differentiating characters." Thus, Mendel provided a way to test for the independent assortment of alleles by analyzing the ratios of offspring of "hybrid" parents who were heterozygous (Aa) for the genotype.

Mendel's second law is referred to as the independent segregation of genes. Generally, the alleles at one of the parents' genes segregate independently of the alleles at another locus. In Mendel's experience, the transmission of the gene for the texture of the seeds, rough or smooth, did not influence the transmission of the gene for the color of the seeds. Mendel stated the second law this way (page 331):

the offspring of the hybrids in which several essentially different characters are combined exhibit the terms of a series of combinations, in which the developmental series for each pair of differentiating characters are united. It is demonstrated at the same time that the relation of each pair of different characters in hybrid union is independent of the other differences in the two original parental stocks.

The independent segregation of genes could be assessed by analyzing the ratios for the various combinations of characters that could be predicted. As developed by Mendel and his intellectual heirs, the early science of genetics was the analysis of transmission ratios following breeding of individuals of known or presumed genetic makeup.

Mendelism, in its own terms, is dependent upon the vagaries of statistical outcomes and the imprecision of human observation. Large numbers of progeny need to be studied in order to be certain about the transmission ratios, but even then the assignment of the progeny may not be accurate. The traits that Mendel analyzed, rough and smooth, yellow and green, are not quite so discreet and could be subject to observer bias. Nonetheless, William Bateson perceived that the laws of genetic transmission provided a material basis for understanding human variation and disease. In his book, *Mendel's Principles of Heredity,* Bateson suggested that if the parents were studied carefully their contributions to their offspring could be discerned.[9] Yet, when applied to humans, Mendelism was problematical because most human matings do not result in large numbers of offspring. Furthermore, many of the more discrete obvious human traits, eye color, hair color, and height, do not demonstrate simple transmission ratios.

As a result, Mendelism in humans was first demonstrated for unusual traits, or rare diseases—among them, short hands (brachydactyly),[10] blood in the urine (hereditary hematuria or Alport syndrome),[11] recurrent nose bleeds or bleeding in the urine, stools, or lungs (hereditary hemorrhagic telangiectasia or Osler-Rendu-Weber disease),[12] thickened palms and soles *(keratosis palmaris et plantaris),*[13] irregular heart beat (familial heart block),[14] and jaundice (Gilbert syndrome).[15] These early studies highlighted the utility of studying rare conditions in humans but also led to the belief that Mendelism might apply only to rare conditions.

On the heels of Mendel's rediscovery were some observations that highlighted exceptions to his rules. The first exception was sex-linked inheritance, a concept that was developed from studies of the fruit fly, drosophila. Sex-linked generally indicated that males had a phenotype more commonly than females. In 1911, E.B. Wilson demonstrated that color blindness was sex-linked.[16] This could be explained by the males having only one copy of the gene for the phenotype, whereas the females had two copies. Both the frequency of color blindness and its transmission could be explained if affected males had one loss-of-function gene (and no normal copy), whereas affected females had two copies. Females who had one loss-of-function gene and a second, normal copy, were "carriers" who could have affected sons but were themselves unaffected.

The second exception to Mendel's laws, linkage, was also found within a short span of time of their rediscovery. Thomas Hunt Morgan and his co-workers observed that some genes in drosophila do not segregate.[17] Rather, because these genes are physically linked to one another on chromosomes, they tend to be transmitted together. Linkage was found to be applicable to humans. Linkage in humans was first demonstrated by Julia Bell and J.B.S. Haldane, who showed that in some families, hemophilia and color blindness tended to be inherited together rather than segregating independently.[18] These two exceptions, linkage and sex-linked inheritance, showed that testing for Mendelian ratios may not be sufficient to identify the genetic basis of human phenotypes.

THE METHODS OF THE GENETICIST

The science of genetics that was developed by Mendel and his successors used mating as a tool to examine the transmission of physical traits. The human geneticist frequently asks what caused an individual to have a specific phenotype. Because the human geneticist cannot control mating, other methods were developed to identify the genetic basis of human traits. The first were methods for precise identification of phenotypes and of patterns of inheritance. Subsequent methods included linkage and association to known genetic traits and markers, analysis of twins, and epidemiological studies.

Phenotype identification. Continuously distributed traits, such as height and serum cholesterol concentrations, while genetically determined, do not commonly show Mendelian transmission. Rather, outliers of such phenotypes, including familial dwarfism and familial hypercholesterolemia, demonstrate Mendelian transmission in some families. The demonstration of Mendelian transmission has also been successful for discontinuous qualitative phenotypes such as color blindness and blood groups.

Similar phenotypes can have different causes, which often can be discerned by careful examination. For example, there are many different causes of familial dwarfism. The presentation is similar, but the cause (different genes) differs. To help decide on the diagnosis, it is necessary to determine the degree of involvement of different bone groups (long bones, spines, and skull and facial bones), the region of the bone that is affected (epiphysis, metaphysis, or diaphysis), and the elements of bone that are involved (calcium, connective tissue, and complex sugar groups known as mucopolysaccharides). Likewise, to help pinpoint the cause it is important to examine the involvement of nonskeletal organs, including eyes, ears, and brain.

A similar strategy is used to discern the different forms of muscular dystrophy. To help make the diagnosis, the affected muscle groups (facial, trunk, limb—both proximal and distal) and muscle fibers (type I and type II) are identified, as is the rate of progression of the disease.

Phenotypic analysis can have two major limitations. First, the classification has not always been rigorous. Distinctions that seem obvious today were missed in the past.[19] Second, there has been much debate about whether conditions with overlapping phenotypes or varying severity represent the same or different entities ("lumping or splitting"). Often these issues cannot be resolved until the disease locus is mapped, or even cloned. This presents a major difficulty because accurate diagnosis is itself critical for gene mapping and cloning.

The catalog for phenotypes is Victor McKusick's *Mendelian Inheritance in Man,* originally published in 1964, and now updated on a continuous basis in an online version. Currently, the catalog lists over 7,000 conditions, which represent distinct phenotypes or allelic forms for some conditions.[20] The frequency of single gene disorders in North America has been tracked by the British Columbia Birth Defects Registry. The overall frequency is estimated to be 1%, with 0.7% as dominant conditions, 0.25% as recessive conditions and 0.04% as X-linked conditions.[21]

Using McKusick's catalog as a guide, the impact of disadaptive Mendelian phenotypes in humans has been examined.[22] Of these, 25% are apparent at birth and over 90% by the end of puberty. Conditions with decreased reproductive fitness generally are manifested earlier in life. Generally, disadaptive Mendelian phenotypes require that some cumulative damage occur before they are apparent. Over half of the phenotypes involve more than one anatomic or functional system. Lifespan is reduced in 57% of these disorders, more commonly in autosomal recessive and X-linked diseases. In 69% of disorders, reproductive capacity is reduced. The nervous system is affected in over 30% of disorders. The age of appearance tends to be more variable for autosomal dominant than for autosomal recessive or X-linked. These studies of frequency, morbidity, and fitness of single-gene conditions were based on known human disorders. These figures may represent an underestimate, because the Mendelian basis for fetal and adult-onset disorders may not have been recognized when these studies were performed.

Segregation analysis. Segregation analysis demonstrates that phenotypic traits are inherited with predictable ratios. The methods for segregation analysis are based on Bateson's dictum, "If the parents differ in several characteristics, the offspring must be examined statistically, and marshaled, as it is called, in respect to each of those characteristics separately."[9] Three patterns of single-gene transmission are recognized in humans, autosomal dominant, autosomal recessive, and X-linked. To demonstrate that the observed patterns of transmission are not due to random chance, statistical goodness-of-fit methods have been developed to rigorously analyze the transmission ratios in families.

Autosomes are any of the 22 pairs of chromosomes that do not show sex-linked transmission. Autosomal dominant traits are generally expressed in the heterozygous state (Fig. 1.1). (An apparent exception occurs with certain inherited cancer genes, discussed in chapter 4). The likelihood of transmitting a dominant trait from parents to children is usually 50%. Generally they are expressed equally in males and females. Dominant genetic traits as described by Mendel in peas and Morgan and his co-workers in drosophila are phenotypically indistinguishable in the homozygous or heterozygous state; however, this is not observed frequently in human genetics. Dominant traits, such as familial hypercholesterolemia, may be more severe in the homozygous state.[23] For some traits, including blood groups, hemoglobin variants, and a variety of serum proteins, expression of the allele from each of the parents can be demonstrated, a phenomenon that is termed, *codominance.*

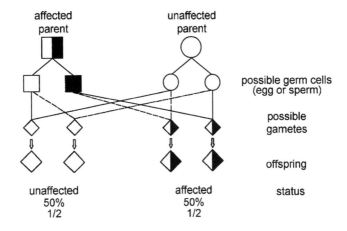

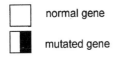

normal gene

mutated gene

Figure 1.1. Pedigree demonstrating autosomal dominant inheritance. The gametes from the affected parent may contain either a normal or a mutated gene. The offspring that are produced from the gamete containing the mutated gene are affected like their parent. The likelihood that an affected parent will have an affected offspring is 50%.

Autosomal recessive traits are generally expressed in homozygotes but not in heterozygotes (Fig. 1.2). Usually the likelihood that carrier parents will have affected offspring is 25%. Because recessive genes are relatively rare, autosomal recessive conditions are found more commonly in ethnic groups who breed among themselves or in families where relatives have married. Proof of this pattern of inheritance requires demonstrating that both parents are heterozygotes. This can be readily accomplished if each of the parental alleles can be identified. For example, as determined by electrophoretic analysis of hemoglobin, β-globin alleles are codominantly expressed. A carrier parent demonstrates expression of one wild-type and one disease allele (e.g., S, C, or D). Alternatively, in some conditions that are expressed when two loss-of-function alleles are present (e.g., reduced enzyme activity) quantifiable reduction in the gene product can be observed frequently in the heterozygous parents. In the absence of a heterozygote detection test, autosomal recessive inheritance cannot be distinguished from other genetic models, including a dominant mutation that has arisen in the germ cells of the transmitting parent.

X-linked conditions are more commonly manifested in males than in females. Because males transmit their Y rather than their X chromosomes to their

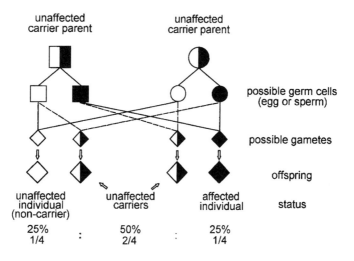

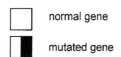

Figure 1.2. Pedigree demonstrating autosomal recessive inheritance. The gametes from the unaffected carrier parents may contain either a normal or a mutated gene. The offspring that are produced from the gametes containing mutated genes from both parents are affected with the disorder. The offspring that are produced from the gametes containing mutated genes from only one parents are carriers like their parents. The offspring that are produced from the gametes containing normal genes from both parents are unaffected, noncarriers. For carrier parents, the likelihood that a child will be affected is 25%. The likelihood that the child will be a carrier is 50%.

sons, X linkage is characterized by the absence of male-to-male transmission (Fig. 1.3). By contrast, all of the daughters of affected males inherit the gene for the condition. Those conditions for which the presence of a single allele is sufficient to result in expression in females are X-linked dominant, whereas those conditions for which two alleles are necessary for expression in females are referred to as X-linked recessive. Relatively few X-linked dominant conditions have been identified. These conditions, hypophosphatemic rickets,[24] fragile X syndrome,[25] and adrenomyeloneuropathy,[26] are generally milder in females than they are in males. Some X-linked dominant conditions, such as incontinentia pigmenti and Rett syndrome,[27,28] are never observed in males and are presumed to be lethal in the absence of two X chromosomes.

Sometimes more than one pattern of inheritance has been found to apply to

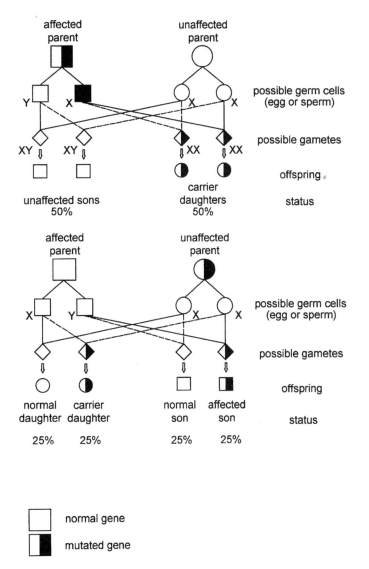

Figure 1.3. Pedigrees demonstrating X-linked inheritance. (A) The X-chromosome-bearing gametes from the affected father contain a mutated gene and the offspring produced from these gametes are carrier females. If this is a dominant disorder, they may be affected. The Y-chromosome-bearing gametes do not have this gene and offspring produced from these gametes are unaffected males. The likelihood that an affected male will have a carrier daughter is 50%. The likelihood that an affected male will have an unaffected son is likewise 50%. (B) The gametes from the carrier mother may contain either a normal or a mutated gene. Depending on the sex chromosome transmitted by the father's gamete, she may have either affected or unaffected sons, and carrier or noncarrier daughters. The likelihood for each of these possible outcomes is 25%.

the development of a phenotypically identical disease state.[29] Retinitis pigmentosa is a condition of progressive vision loss that starts with night blindness. This condition affects approximately one in 40,000 people. Several different patterns of transmission have been observed, including autosomal dominant, autosomal recessive, and X-linked. These findings suggest that mutations in several different genes can produce retinitis pigmentosa. In some families with autosomal dominant retinitis pigmentosa, the mutation is located in the rhodopsin gene on chromosome 3.[30] In other families with autosomal dominant retinitis pigmentosa, the mutation is located in the peripherin gene on chromosome 6[31] or in a gene that has not yet been identified on chromosome 8.[32] Mutations in at least two different genes on the X chromosome account for the X-linked form of this condition.[33] This phenomenon of different genes producing identical phenotypes is known as "genetic locus heterogeneity."

The fact that several individuals within the same family may have the same trait does not prove genetic causality, because individuals within families share environments as well as genes. The trait that is selected for pedigree analysis should reflect a measurable physical attribute in the host; otherwise the analysis may seem trivial. By segregation analysis alone, the choice of profession has been demonstrated to simulate autosomal recessive inheritance.[34] Rigorous proof of genetic transmission requires use of other methods, including linkage to a known genetic trait or marker.

Linkage analysis. Two genes are linked when they are inherited with a frequency greater than the 50% predicted by Mendel's second law (Fig. 1.4). Demonstrating linkage of a phenotype to a marker that is known to show Mendelian transmission is one of the most robust techniques of genetic analysis. Linkage can be demonstrated for genes and markers that lie in in close physical proximity on the same chromosome. As the distance increases between a gene and a series of test markers on a chromosome, the tendency for linkage falls off because the likelihood of chromosomal recombination increases.

Ordinarily, during the process of sperm cell or egg cell development, the two chromosomes in a pair undergo recombination. The farther apart two loci are, the greater the chance that a recombination event will occur between them. When there is recombination between two genes on a chromosome, their linked transmission is disrupted. The frequency with which recombination occurs between the two genes determines the genetic distance between them.

Markers that can be used for linkage analysis include phenotypes, such as color blindness or hemophilia, soluble proteins whose variants can be distinguished electrophoretically, surface proteins whose variants can be distinguished immunologically, and benign chromosomal variants whose variants can be distinguished microscopically. Currently, the most frequently used genetic markers are variations in DNA sequences not causing changes in expression because these tend to show the greatest polymorphism among humans. These tend to be of two types—point mutations and variable number of repeats of short sequences of DNA.

Two criteria are generally required to detect genetic linkage. First, the fre-

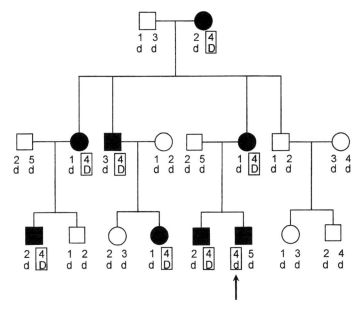

Figure 1.4. Pedigree demonstrating linkage. Affected individuals are shown in black and unaffected individuals are shown in white. The gene for this condition is being transmitted along with the 4 allele at a linked marker locus. Note that a recombination occurred for the individual indicated by the arrow.

quency of polymorphisms in the population should be high, thereby increasing the likelihood of distinguishing the corresponding regions of a given individual's pair of chromosomes. Second, the distance between the marker and the gene of interest should be small. For more tightly linked and polymorphic markers, fewer individuals within a pedigree or fewer pedigrees may need to be studied to demonstrate linkage.

Linkage between a phenotypic trait and a genetic marker or between two genetic markers is generally measured as the logarithm of an odds ratio. This ratio measure the odds of the likelihood that there is linkage at a certain genetic distance to the likelihood that there is no linkage at all. This test is given the name of a LOD score, because it measures the log of the odds.[35] Generally a LOD score of 3 or greater is taken as an indication that linkage exists, because this indicates that odds ratio was 1,000 to one. Under most conditions, this indicates a greater than 95% likelihood that true linkage exists.

Sometimes large families may not be available for performing classical linkage analysis. Alternative methods have been developed that examine for nonrandom sharing of alleles among siblings or other relatives who have the same condition. Generally, the likelihood that two sibs will share two, one, or zero alleles in common at any given locus is 1/4:1/2:1/4. If significant deviation from these ratios is observed for a group of siblings who share the same condition, then this finding is indicative of linkage to that locus. This form of analysis generally requires participation from large numbers of families and has been useful for identifying genes for some common diseases.

In the absence of any clues, several hundred markers may need to be studied in order to establish linkage between the gene for a given trait and at least one genetic marker (and thereby localize the gene for the trait).[36] This process has been facilitated by the concerted efforts of many laboratories to identify highly polymorphic DNA markers. When used to study several large reference families, the distances between these markers have been determined by linkage analysis, thereby generating genetic maps of the human chromosomes.[37] As a result, once an unknown disease gene has been linked to a genetic marker, its position on the genetic map is known. The recombination with markers can be used as a way of refining the position of the disease gene on a chromosome.

Sometimes segregation analysis or fortuitous associations of a disease with other genetic markers can suggest possible locations of a disease gene. For example, the absence of male-to-male transmission for a trait suggests looking for X chromosome linkage. The demonstration that a consistent chromosomal alteration is associated with some cases of a disease suggests the presence of the disease-causing gene in the altered region. For example, some familial cases of retinoblastoma, a tumor of the retina, are associated with deletions of chromosome 13 in the blood and tissues of individuals who develop this condition.[11,38] Based on this observation, familial cases with no demonstrable deletion were analyzed using chromosome 13 markers and linkage was demonstrated, indicating the presence of a disease-causing gene on this chromosome.

Candidate genes that are suspected of causing disease on the basis of their protein products or on the basis of their map location can be tested for linkage to the disease locus. If no recombination is observed between the candidate and the disease locus, the candidate or a gene in close proximity is disease-causing. The demonstration of mutations in affected individuals that are not present in their unaffected relatives strongly suggests that gene causes the disease in question. (This concept is developed further in chapter 2.)

Association. Some conditions have a genetic basis but do not demonstrate Mendelian transmission in families (Fig. 1.5). A genetic basis for these conditions has been demonstrated by association to a specific allele of a genetic marker in people with the phenotype at a greater frequency than would be predicted by chance alone. Generally, the frequency of the marker in the unaffected population is too high for it to be a sufficient cause of the condition. Rather, the presence of this marker increases the likelihood for developing the condition.

The best-known examples of genetic associations are those between human leukocyte antigen (HLA) alleles that play a role in the regulation of the immune system and autoimmune disorders. These conditions, including ankylosing spondylitis, rheumatoid arthritis, and insulin-dependent diabetes mellitus, result when the activity of the immune system is directed against the body's own tissues. In ankylosing spondylitis, a degenerative disorder of the spine and other joints, 92% of individuals with the condition have at least one HLA B27 al-

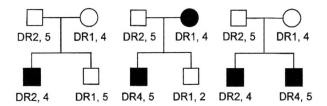

Figure 1.5. Pedigrees demonstrating associations (independent of linkage). Affected individuals are shown in black and unaffected individuals are shown in white. The 4 allele is found in almost all affected and some unaffected individuals in these pedigrees regardless of the apparent pattern of transmission.

lele.[39] Most cases of rheumatoid arthritis and insulin-dependent diabetes mellitus are associated commonly with HLA-DR3 or DR4.[40,41] Based on the function of HLA loci, it has been inferred that the immune response of the hosts may vary compared to those who do not have these alleles. The alternative hypothesis is that the HLA allele does not cause the disease, but the HLA allele is associated with the disease-causing allele of another gene. This hypothesis has not been excluded.

Association differs from linkage because individuals, rather than families, are studied. As a result, transmission of susceptibility is not being demonstrated. The robustness of association as a technique has been augmented by the use of multiple linked markers. If the association to a given chromosomal region is not fortuitous, then it can be demonstrated for alleles for each of the markers that is being analyzed. The strength of the association is greater for markers that are closer to the susceptibility gene. Stronger associations are observed in small, isolated populations with a founder effect. This occurs because the number of alleles producing a specific phenotype is smaller in such populations and the number of generations since the occurrence of such alleles tends to be small. As a result, the genetic association may extend for some distance over a chromosome.

Twin studies. Analyzing twins for the presence of a specific phenotype is another way to demonstrate a genetic basis for conditions that seem to be clustered in families.[42,43] Monozygotic twins are derived from the same zygote and thus inherit the same genetic constitution. By contrast, dizygotic twins share only half of their genes in common on average. Both types of twins share a common uterine environment during gestational life and frequently share a common rearing environment; thus, the demonstration of a higher degree of concordance for a trait in monozygotic twins compared to dizygotic twins is generally taken as evidence that a trait is genetically encoded. This does not provide an indication for the pattern of inheritance for the trait. The fact that monozygotic twins may be discordant for genetically encoded traits suggests that factors in addition to genetic inheritance may be at work. To test for the role of the environment in the development of these traits, some studies take advantage of the fact that twins may be adopted individually at birth and reared in different environments. A high concordance rate has been observed for many behavioral traits among monozygotic twins who were reared apart. These findings have suggested that genes contribute to the development of behavior.

Epidemiological studies. Epidemiological studies have been used to identify factors that predispose to specific human phenotypes.[44] Currently, these studies tend to include identification of environmental factors, such as infectious agents or toxins, and identification of an underlying host factor that confers susceptibility, often on a genetic basis. Such host factors may include receptors or a rate-limiting enzyme in a metabolic pathway.

FACTORS INFLUENCING GENE FREQUENCIES IN HUMAN POPULATIONS

The unique makeup of each person is determined by his or her genetic constitution, that is, the specific genes that were transmitted to that person by the parents. In turn, the parents' genetic constitutions were influenced by the populations from which they originated. Such populations may be small and marry within their own membership, or large and have no preferences regarding mating. The frequency of specific alleles of various genes in a population is highly variable—from a single occurrence to being the most predominant form in the population (Fig. 1.6). Other factors also influence the frequencies of genes in populations.

Mutation. One factor is the mutation rate in germ cells that drives the formation of new alleles. The mutation rate in germ cells has been calculated to be around 10^{-5} to 10^{-4} for neurofibromatosis I, tuberous sclerosis, and retinoblastoma.[45-47] The rate of mutation has been postulated to be correlated with the size of the gene. Another factor influencing mutation rates is instability in a gene. (This topic is developed in greater detail in chapter 8.)

Fitness and selection. Another factor that influences the frequency of alleles in populations is the genetic fitness of the individuals who carry those alleles, that is, the ability of individuals who inherit the alleles to survive and reproduce, passing the allele on to future generations. The fitness can vary for different alleles from having minimal effect to completely eliminating the ability to reproduce. Most new mutations reduce the fitness of their carriers and thus are selected against. For some dominant diseases in which the fitness is very low, most of the cases represent new mutations.

The counterpart to genetic fitness in a population is selection. Selection may occur for alleles that increase genetic fitness in the presence of certain environments. In populations from many regions of the world, selection for resistance to falciparum malaria has caused the frequency of hemoglobinopathy (i.e., hemoglobin S, C, D, and E), thalassemia and glucose-6-phosphate deficiency alleles to become very high.[48] This has occurred despite the deleterious conse-

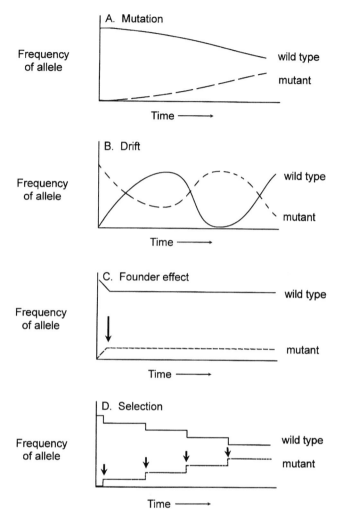

Figure 1.6. Factors influencing gene frequencies are: (A). *Mutation:* As the result of new mutations, the frequency of mutant alleles increases in the population. (B) *Drift:* As the result of chance alone (generally in a small population), the frequency of the mutant allele varies over time. Such alleles may become fixed or eliminated. (C) *Founder effect:* As the result of the introduction of a mutation into a population by a founder (indicated by the arrow), the frequency of the mutant allele increased. (D) *Selection:* As the result of a series of selection events (indicated by the arrows), the frequency of the mutant allele has increased over time.

quences of being homozygous for the disease gene, because the ability of heterozygotes to reproduce is higher than that of normal (or diseased) homozygotes. For some disease alleles with a high population frequency, a heterozygote advantage has been presumed, but the basis for this advantage is unclear.

Genetic drift and founder effects. Some alleles are selectively neutral and their fates are determined by other forces. One force is genetic drift, in which differences in allelic frequencies occur as the result of chance fluctuations. The magnitude of such fluctuations is greater in small populations than in large. Another force is the founder effect. One, or a few, individuals introduce a new allele into a small inbreeding population. In time, the frequency of this allele may become greater in this population than in the population in which the mutation originated. Founder effects are presumed to have caused the frequencies of tyrosinemia and Ellis van Creveld syndrome to be high, respectively, among in French Canadians in northern Quebec and the Amish in the Pennsylvania.[49,50]

Gene frequencies within any population are balanced by chance variation on the one hand and by selection for specific alleles on the other. There are several ways to distinguish among these possibilities. First, the historical record may indicate whether the population migrated or suffered a severe reduction in the number of its young members. Second, for recessive disorders, the number of living heterozygotes may be greater and the number of homozygotes less than would be predicted. These findings would suggest selection for heterozygotes and against homozygotes. Third, mutations in the population may be associated with specific alleles of linked markers, suggesting that the mutation occurred one or a limited number of times in the population.

Identification of the laws of transmission and of a series of methods for demonstrating genetic associations represented the first steps for understanding the genetic basis of human variation. The next steps required an understanding of how genes work, both in the normal and abnormal states.

REFERENCES

1. Mendel G. Versuche über Pflanzen-Hybriden. Ver Natur Vere Brü 4:3–47, 1865. English translation by Royal Hort. Soc. London., Harvard Univ. Press, 1916.
2. Correns C. 'G. Mendel's Regel über das Verhalten der Nachkommenschaft der Rassenbastarde. Ber Deut Botan Gessel 18:158–168, 1900.
3. De Vries H. Sur la loi de disjonction des hybrides. Acad Sci Paris 130:845–847, 1900.
4. Tschermak E. Uber kunstliche Kreuzung bei Pisum sativum. Zeit landw Versuch n Oest 3:465–555, 1900.
5. Fisher RA. 'The correlation between relatives on the supposition of Mendelian inheritance. Trans R Soc Edinb 52:399–433, 1918.
6. Sturtevant AH. A History of Genetics. New York: Harper and Row, 1965.
7. Dunn L.C. A Short History of Genetics. New York: McGraw-Hill, 1965.
8. Diamond B, Chien N, Scharff M. Somatic mutation alters affinity and specificity. Ann Inst Pasteur Immunol 136C:267–271, 1985.
9. Bateson W. Mendel's Principles of Heredity. London: Cambridge University Press, 1909.
10. Bauer B. Eine bisher nicht beobachtete kongenitale, hereditaere Anomalie des Fingerskelettes. Dtsch Z Chir 86:252–259, 1907.

11. Wilson MG, Towner JW, Fujimoto A. Retinoblastoma and D-chromosome deletions. Anr J Hum Genet 25:57–61, 1973.

12. Osler W. On a family form of recurring epistaxis associated with multiple telangiectases of the skin and mucous membranes. Johns Hopkins Hosp Bull 7:333–337, 1901.

13. Vorner H. Zur Kenntniss der Keratoma hereditarium palmare et plantare. Arch Dermatol Syph 56:3–31, 1901.

14. Morguio L. Sur une maladie infantile et familiale caracterisee par des modifications permanentes du pouls,des attaques syncopales et epileptiformes et la mort subite. Arch Med Enfants 4:467–475, 1901.

15. Gilbert A, Lereboullet P. La cholemie simple familiale. Semaine Med 21:241–243, 1901.

16. Wilson EB. The sex chromosomes. Arch Mikrosk Anat Enwicklungsmech 77:249–271, 1911.

17. Morgan TH, Sturtevant AH, Muller HJ, Bridges CB. The Mechanism of Mendelian Inheritance. New York: Henry Holt, 1915.

18. Bell J, Haldane JBS. The linkage between the genes for color-blindness and haemophilia in men. Proc R Soc Lond [Biol] 123:119–150, 1937.

19. Harper PS. Myotonic Dystrophy. Philadelphia: WB Saunders, 1989.

20. McKusick VA. Mendelian Inheritance in Man. 8th ed. Baltimore: Johns Hopkins University Press, 1988.

21. Baird PA, Anderson TW, Newcombe HB, Lowry RB. Genetic disorders in children and young adults: a population study. Am J Hum Genet 42:677–693, 1988.

22. Costa T, Scriver CR, Childs B. The effect of Mendelian disease on human health: a measurement. Am J Med Genet 21:231,1985.

23. Brown MS, Goldstein JL. A receptor-mediated pathway for cholesterol homeostasis. Science 232:34–47, 1986.

24. Winters RW, Graham JB, Williams TF, McFalls VW, Burnett CH. A genetic study of familial hypophosphatemia and vitamin D-resistant rickets with a review of the literature. Medicine 37:97–142, 1958.

25. Loesch DZ, Hay DA. Clinical features and reproductive patterns in fragile X female heterozygotes. J Med Genet 25:407–414, 1988.

26. Moser HW, Moser AE, Singh I, O'Neill BP. Adrenoleukodystrophy: survey of 303 cases: biochemistry, diagnosis, and therapy. Ann Neurol 16:628–641, 1984.

27. Lenz W. Zur Genetik der Incontinentia pigmenti. Ann Paediat 196:149–165, 1961.

28. Comings DE. The genetics of Rett syndrome: the consequences of a disorder where every case is a new mutation. Am J Med Genet Suppl 1:383–388, 1986.

29. Humphries P, Kenna P, Farrar GJ. On the molecular genetics of retinitis pigmentosa. Science 256:804–808, 1992.

30. McWilliams P, Farrar GJ, Kenna P, Bradley DG, Humphries MM, Sharp EM, et al. Autosomal dominant retinitis pigmentosa (ADRP): localization of an ADRP gene to the long arm of chromosome 3. Genomics 5:619–622, 1989.

31. Jordan SA, Farrar GJ, Kumar-Singh R, Kenna P, Humphries MM, Allamand V, et al. Autosomal dominant retinitis pigmentosa (adRP; RP6): cosegregation of RP6 and the peripherin-RDS locus in a late-onset family of Irish origin. Am J Hum Genet 50:634–639, 1992.

32. Blanton SH, Heckenlively JR, Cottingham AW, Friedman J, Sadler LA, Wagner M, et al. Linkage mapping of autosomal dominant retinitis pigmentosa (RPI) to the pericentric region of human chromosome 8. Genomics 11:857–869, 1991.

33. Chen J-D, Halliday F, Keith G, Sheffield L, Dickinson P, Gray R, et al. Linkage heterogeneity between X-linked retinitis pigmentosa and a map of 10 RFLP loci. Am J Hum Genet 45:401–411, 1989.

34. McGuffin P, Huckle P. Simulation of Mendelism revisited: the recessive gene for attending medical school. Am J Hum Genet 46:994–999, 1990.

35. Morton NE. The detection and estimation of linkage between the genes for elliptocytosis and the Rh blood type. Am J Hum Genet 8:80–96, 1956.

36. Botstein D, White RL, Skolnick M, Davis RW. Construction of a genetic linkage map in man using restriction fragment length polymorphisms. Am J Hum Genet 32:314–331, 1980.

37. National Research Council. Mapping and Sequencing the Human Genome. Washington, DC: National Academy of Sciences, 1988.

38. Gey W. Dq-, multiple Missbildungen und Retinoblastom. Humgenetik 10:362–365, 1970.

39. Schlosstein L, Terasaki PI, Bluestone R, Pearson CM. High association of an HL-A antigen,W27,with ankylosing spondylitis. New Engl J Med 288:704–706, 1973.

40. Stastny P, Fink CW. Different HLA-D associations in adult and juvenile rhuematoid arthritis. J Clin Invest 63:124–130, 1979.

41. Rotter JI, Rimoin DL. Diabetes mellitus: the search for genetic markers. Diabetes Care 2:215–216, 1979.

42. Becker KL. The twin-study method in medicine and genetics. Postgrad Med 41:603–608, 1967.

43. Nance WE. The role of twin studies in human quantitative genetics. Prog Med Genet 3:73–107, 1979.

44. Motulsky AG. Genetic epidemiology. Genet Epidemiol 1:143–144, 1984.

45. Crowe JF, Schull WJ, Neel JV. A clinical,pathological,and genetic study of multiple neurofibromatosis. Springfield: Thomas, 1956.

46. Vogel F. Neue Untersuchungen zur Genetik des Retinoblastoms (Glioma retinae). Z Menschl Vererbun -Konstitu 34:205–236, 1957.

47. Ohno K, Takeshita K, Arima M. Frequency of tuberous sclerosis in San-in district (Japan) and birth weight of patients with tuberous sclerosis. Brain Dev 3:57–64, 1981.

48. Friedman MJ, Trager W. The biochemistry of resistance to malaria. Sci Am 244:154–164, 1981.

49. Bergeron P, Labarge C, Grenier A. Hereditary tyrosinemia in the province of Quebec: prevalence at birth and geographic distribution. Clin Genet 5:157–162, 1974.

50. McKusick VA, Egeland JA, Eldridge R, Krusen DR. Dwarfism in the Amish. I. The Ellis-van Creveld syndrome. Johns Hopkins Hosp Bull 115:306, 1964.

2

The Molecular Basis of Mendelian Disease

Our understanding of the molecular basis of genetic disease was developed by identifying mutations in genes that showed Mendelian transmission and the effects of these mutations on the encoded polypeptides. Thus we learned that disease occurs when an anatomic or physiological system is disrupted in such a way that the individual cannot mount a sufficient compensatory response. Initially it was thought that all mutations knocked out the functions of a gene. Subsequently, it was learned that mutations may alter the stability of the gene product or confer novel functions on that product. The molecular basis of genetic disease instructs not only on the functions of genes but also on the mechanisms by which genetic variation occurs and on the physiology of the system that is disrupted.

ORGANIZATION AND VARIATION IN THE HUMAN GENOME

Organization. Genes are encoded on molecules of deoxyribonucleic acid (DNA) in the nucleus of the cell. Avery and McCarty demonstrated that genes were comprised of DNA molecules. They based their demonstration on the fact that the phenotype was dependent on the specific DNA taken up by the test strains of bacteria. In 1953, Watson and Crick suggested that DNA is composed of two antiparallel strands.[1] Each strand is made up of a linear array of nucleotide bases (the pyrimidines, thymidine and cytidine, and the purines, adenosine and guanosine) that are joined by phosphodiester bonds. The two strands anneal to one another by hydrogen bonding between complementary bases, thymidine and adenosine or cytidine and guanosine. The complementary nature of the two strands provides for faithful replication of the DNA molecule in the nuclei of germ and somatic cells.

The amount of DNA in the haploid human genome is 3×10^9 base pairs of DNA.[2] That would stretch approximately two meters if every molecule were joined together. The DNA is packaged in 46 chromosomes; each chromosome contains a single DNA molecule. In each chromosome, the DNA is wound around histone molecules and further condensed by associations with other proteins that create solenoids and higher order structures. The state of condensation of the DNA varies during the cell cycle; the highest degree of condensation occurs during metaphase, just prior to cell division.

Only 3% of the human genome contains genes.[3] The genes include the regions that encode proteins or structural RNA molecules, noncoding intervening sequences (or introns), and flanking regions that contain sequences that affect the regulation of the genes (Fig. 2.1). Some of the noncoding sequences serve specialized functions. These include sites for chromosomal attachment to the nuclear scaffold,[4,5] sites to initiate DNA replication, and specialized structures at the ends of chromosomes ("telomeres") that prevent attachment to free bits of DNA in the cell.[6,7] The function of the remainder of the genome is unknown. Although not yet demonstrated, specialized sequences may play a role in DNA condensation, recombination, and binding to microtubules during cell division. Much of the DNA appears not to serve a function dependent on its precise sequence. Some of the DNA may not provide functions for the host at all and may act as a parasite within the cell ("selfish DNA").[8-10] Among the DNA sequnces that do not code for proteins are the L1 middle repetitive sequences (~5000 copies per genome) and the Alu highly repetitive sequences (~300,000 copies genome).[11,12]

The DNA in the human genome includes some sequences that are unique and others that are repeated: The repeats range from a few copies to thousands or hundreds of thousands of copies.[2,13] As a result, some products are encoded by single genes, whereas others are encoded by gene families. Among the prod-

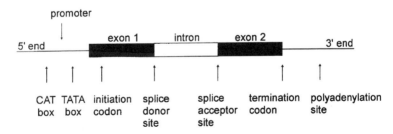

Figure 2.1. Structure of a gene demonstrating the expressed regions *(exons)* and intervening sequences *(introns)* and the 5' and 3' untranscribed regions. Transcription starts at the promoter. The CAT and TATA boxes play a role in the promoter activity. Regions in the transcript include the splice donor and acceptor and polyadenylation sites and the initiator and terminator codons.

ucts of these gene families are ribosomal RNA,[14] histones,[15] globins,[16] colla-gens,[17] and keratins.[18,19] These products serve similar or identical functions. For the α-globin,[16] and ribosomal RNA genes,[20] the sequences of the genes are virtually identical among different members of the gene family. Among the different classes of histones, the sequences of the genes have diverged, but the amino acid sequences of the different members within a class of histone genes have been maintained.[21]

Sometimes different members of a gene family may have diverged suffi-ciently to encode gene products with different functions. For example, the growth hormone gene complex on chromosome 17 includes the genes for growth hormone, a pituitary hormone that promotes protein synthesis and growth, prolactin, a pituitary hormone that stimulates production of milk by the mammary glands, and human chorionic somatomammotropin, a placental hormone whose function has not been identified.[22–24] The photoreceptor pro-teins, rhodopsin and the cone opsins, and the receptors for the nerve cell trans-mitters, acetylcholine epinephrine, norepinephrine, and dopamine, share a com-mon structure with regions that traverse the cell membrane seven times and initiate their signals through interaction with a protein that binds guanosine triphosphatase (GTP).[25–27] The sequences of the receptors have diverged, so their effects are triggered by binding different molecules. Other gene families, including the serpin family of protease inhibitors (α-1-antitrypsin and anti-thrombin III),[28] the immunoglobulin superfamily, which includes the T-cell re-ceptor and HLA genes,[29] and the serum proteins albumin and α-fetoprotein,[30] have also been generated by gene duplication and sequence divergence.

For genes that encode protein molecules, the intermediate signal in the trans-mission of genetic information is messenger RNA (mRNA).[31] The mRNA mol-ecule is transcribed as a complementary sequence from the DNA of a gene by the enzyme RNA polymerase (Fig. 2.2).[32,33] DNA sequences both inside and outside the coding region of the gene regulate the transcription through binding various protein factors.[34] These binding proteins may change the topographical structure of the DNA and may interact with the polymerase. Once transcribed, the mRNA intermediate undergoes a series of modifications that may include deletion of sequences at the 3' end with subsequent addition of adenine residues ("polyadenylation"),[35] splicing of noncoding intervening sequences ("in-trons"),[36] and addition of a methylated guanine to the 5' end ("capping").[37,38]

The mature RNA molecule is transported from the nucleus to the cytoplasm, where it serves as a template for translation into proteins on polysomes. On the polysomes, transfer RNA (tRNA) molecules charged with amino acids bind their triplet codons to the mRNA molecule.[39–41] A peptide bond is formed be-tween the initiating amino acid and the subsequent amino acid.[42–44] This process continues until a termination codon is encountered and translation stops.[45–49] The immature protein molecule ("polypeptide") may undergo a se-ries of posttranslational changes, including cleavage, assembly with the same or other polypeptide molecules, and covalent and noncovalent binding of non-polypeptide molecules.[50–52]

Each of the steps in the transmission of the signal from gene to polypeptide

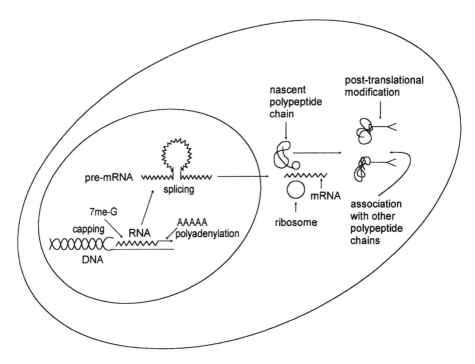

Figure 2.2. Genetic processing demonstrating transcription of a gene. Following transcription, the RNA is capped with 7-methylguanine, polyadenylated, spliced, and transported from the nucleus to the cytoplasm. The cytoplasmic mRNA is translated on ribosomes. The resulting polypeptides may undergo posttranslational modifications and association with other polypeptide chains.

represents an opportunity for genetic control. Variation in the sequence of a gene alters both the accuracy and efficiency with which the steps of RNA processing and translation and posttranslational processing of polypeptides occur. If sequence variation occurs in genes that affect the transmission of information by other genes (for example, transfer RNA), multiple gene products may be affected.

Sequence variation. Sequence variation occurs both within and around genes. Sequence variation within a gene is more likely to affect the function of the gene and thus the phenotype of the organism. Because of this alteration in phenotype, variation within genes may be subject to selection. Sequence variation outside of coding or regulatory regions may not be subject to the same degree of selection. As a result, a higher rate of sequence polymorphism is observed in the flanking regions and in the introns.[53]

The frequency of sequence variation in the human genome has been estimated using several different methods.[54,55] Each method suggests a frequency of nucleotide differences between 0.1 and 1.0%.[56,57] Similar methods have been used to estimate the frequency of sequence variation among the higher primate species. The frequency of sequence variation between humans and chimpanzees or humans and gorillas is similar to the frequency of sequence variation among humans; thus, the speciation of the higher primates is not related to major changes in DNA sequence.[58] Instead, the differences among these species appear to be related to changes in the expression and function of individual genes.[59]

THE MECHANISMS OF MUTATION

Mutation results from a rearrangement in the DNA molecule. These alterations include point mutations, deletions, insertions, unequal recombination, and translocation of DNA (Fig. 2.3).

Point mutations. Point mutations have been observed to be of two types— transitions from one pyrimidine or purine to another, and transversions, changing from a pyrimidine to a purine or vice versa. The overall rate of mutation depends on both the frequency with which mutations occur and the frequency with which they are corrected in the genome. Some regions of the human genome are hotspots for mutation. One hotspot occurs at the base cytosine when it occurs in the CG dinucleotide.[60,61] When methylated, this base is subject to deamination, resulting in a thymine base. This transition also appears to be less efficiently repaired than other types of mutations. In the factor IX gene, the frequency of transitions at the CG site is 24-fold greater than the frequency of other transitions.[57] As a result of this high frequency of transitions in the human genome, the representation of CG dinucleotide is some fivefold less than would be predicted by chance alone.[62]

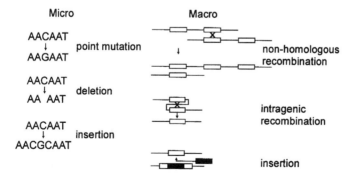

Figure 2.3. Mechanisms of mutation. Mutations may occur on a micro scale affecting one or a few bases and may include substitutions, deletions, or insertions. Mutations may also occur on a macro scale and may include nonhomologous or intragenic recombination and insertion.

Deletions. Deletion of a gene is another commonly observed mutation. Small deletions occur from errors in the replication of genes. Deletions may occur as the result of recombination between similar (but not identical) regions on two chromosomes or on a single chromosome with loss of the intervening fragment. Such unequal recombination has been commonly observed when there has been duplication of an ancestral gene resulting in a gene complex that occurs in a tandem array. In the α-globin gene complex, most human chromosomes have two copies of identical α-globin genes. Through unequal recombination, chromosomes are generated that have one or three copies of the α-globin genes.[63,64]

Deletion can occur within a gene as the result of pairing and recombination of homologous regions. Recombination between the highly repeated Alu sequences has been observed in the low-density-lipoprotein (LDL)-receptor gene, resulting in truncated or defective receptors.[65] Unequal recombination between the δ- and β-globin genes on chromosome 11 resulted in the formation of a hybrid gene, termed "hemoglobin Lepore," containing the 5' end of δ and the 3' end of β with deletion of the genetic sequences in between, the first hybrid protein of this sort to be identified.[66]

Insertion. Short inserts into genes are likely to result from errors in replication. Longer inserts result from a break in a gene with the addition of another DNA molecule. Insertion of the moderately repeated L1 sequence into the factor VIII gene has been observed in at least four cases of hemophilia A.[67] The similarity of these repetitive sequences to transposable elements in other organisms suggests that these sequences are replicated and then transposed from other sites in the human genome.

ORIGIN OF MUTATIONS

Paternal effect. In 1955, Lionel Penrose, an English geneticist, inferred that the rate of new mutations was greater in the germ cells of the father than in those of the mother because of the larger number of cell divisions that take place in male germ cells. His hypothesis was supported by the association of many new dominant mutations with increased paternal age.[68–70] Subsequently, this hypothesis was supported by detailed study of the origin of new hemophilia B mutations in the factor IX gene using linked genetic markers to identify the parental origin of new mutations.[57] Single-base substitutions occurred in the male germ line with a 3.5-fold predominance over female. Transitions at CG dinucleotides were 11-fold more predominant in males, indicating that these sites were hotspots of mutation in male germ cells. Inversion in the factor VIII gene has been associated with almost half the cases of hemophilia A.[57,71] Virtually all of the new occurrences of this mutation have been in male germ cells.[46,72] Unlike dominant and X-linked disorders, new mutations have been rarely identified for autosomal recessive disorders.[73] This is because they only cause phenotypic changes in an individual with two mutated copies of the gene.

Genetic background. Through analysis of linked marker alleles, it is possible to infer the origin of a mutation within a population.[74,75] The mutation may be associated with a single allele at a closely linked marker locus, suggesting that the mutation arose on a chromosome that contained that marker allele. Mutations that are associated with multiple alleles at the marker locus may have occurred in at least one of two different ways. First, the mutation may have arisen multiple times, once on each of these different genetic backgrounds. Alternatively, the mutation may have become associated with the different markers by recombination between the mutated gene and the marker. From knowledge of the rate of mutation and the rate of recombination between the marker and the mutation, the likelihood that the mutation arose several times can be calculated.

Based on this approach, it has been demonstrated that the major recessive mutations in geographically isolated, inbreeding populations had a single origin (e.g., idiopathic torsion dystonia in Ashkenazi Jews,[76] diastrophic dysplasia among Finns,[77] and Friedreich ataxia among Louisiana Acadians[78]). Common recessive mutations among populations that were neither inbreeding nor geographically isolated had multiple origins. For example, the hemoglobin S mutation among people of African descent[79] and the common European phenylketonuria mutation (glutamine to lysine at codon 280 of the phenylalanine hydroxylase gene) are found on chromosomes with multiple different marker alleles, suggesting that they arose more than once.[80]

This approach has been used in a prospective manner to predict the number of disease alleles for a given gene. Although a disease gene might not have been identified, one or a few alleles of the marker can show nonrandom association with the disease locus. The number of such marker allele associations may be predictive of the number of disease alleles. In addition, the frequency with which these markers occur in disease allele-bearing chromosomes may be indicative of the relative frequencies of the disease alleles themselves.

THE EFFECTS OF MUTATION

Mutations produce phenotypic effects by altering the quantity of gene product or the function of this product (Fig. 2.4). Thalassemia is a disorder in which there is quantitative reduction in globin chains.[81] In ß-thalassemia, the disorder is linked to the β-globin gene complex, demonstrating that the defect is intrinsic to the β-globin gene itself. Indeed, many different mutations in the β-globin gene affect the transcription, splicing, or translation of the mRNA and reduce the production of β-globin polypeptide. In most populations at risk, no single mutation accounts for most of the β-thalassemia alleles. As a result, most cases of disease are associated with compound heterozygosity (a different mutation on each of the two chromosomes, rather than with homozygosity for a single mutation).

Mutations can alter the activity of a protein. Mutations that affect the active sites of enzymes can decrease the efficiency of the reaction that is catalyzed by

Wild type

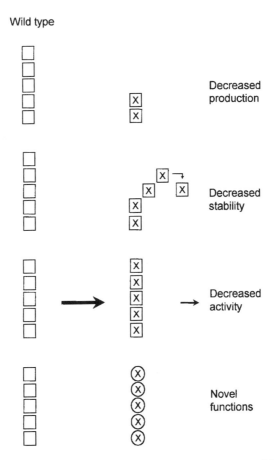

Figure 2.4. Mutation may operate to decrease the production, stability, or activity of a protein, or a mutation may cause a protein to assume novel functions.

the enzyme. This can occur by decreasing the affinity of the enzyme for the substrate or by decreasing the rate of the reaction. For nonenzymatic proteins, mutations can alter the affinity of the protein for its ligand. Mutations in globin genes can increase or decrease the affinity of hemoglobin molecules for oxygen (Hb Hiroshima[82,83] and Hb Kansas,[84,85] respectively). Mutations that diminish the affinity of the insulin- and androgen-receptor proteins for their ligands produce insulin-unresponsive diabetes mellitus with leprechaunism and incomplete virilization of individuals with 46,XY chromosomal constitutions, respectively.[86] Mutations that diminish the affinity of the SRY protein for its DNA binding sites abolish the signal for testicular differentiation, resulting in gonadal dysgenesis.[87,88]

Other intrinsic functions of the protein may be altered. The spectral sensitivity of the X-linked cone opsin visual pigment proteins can be shifted as a result of mutation. If the spectral shift is more than a few nanometers, males who carry these altered genes in the hemizygous state have mild or severe color blindness.[89,90] For proteins such as collagen and keratins that serve a structural role in bones, ligaments, and skin, mutations can alter their ability to form macromolecules, thus resulting in structurally deficient or quantitatively diminished proteins.[91,92]

In some instances molecules with novel functions have been identified as resulting from mutation. The best-known example is the S mutation in the β-globin gene that results from the substitution of a valine for a glutamic acid at residue 6.[93] The effect of this substitution is to cause sickling of hemoglobin S under low oxygen tensions. The effects of the ß[S] mutation can be exacerbated or ameliorated by a second mutation. In HbS[Antilles], the second mutation is the substitution of isoleucine for valine at position 23 of the β-globin gene.[94] Inheritance of a ß[SAntilles] gene is sufficient to cause the manifestations of sickle cell anemia in the heterozygous state.

An unusual example of mutation producing a molecule with altered function has been demonstrated for α-1-antitrypsin. This molecule is a circulating serpin protease inhibitor that acts on elastase. Deficiency of this molecule is associated with emphysema. This protein is an acute phase reactant that increases in response to infection and other stresses. Antithrombin III (AT3) is another member of the serpin family of protease inhibitors. This molecule is an inhibitor of thrombin, preventing the cleavage of fibrinogen to form fibrin, thus preventing clotting. In one individual with an unusual point mutation, the active site of the α-1-antitrypsin molecule was converted from methionine to arginine, thus making it function as an antithrombin III molecule. In response to acute phase stimuli, the increased production of the genetically altered α-1-antitrypsin resulted in a severe bleeding disorder.[95]

Some mutations alter the stability, but not the function, of the polypeptides. When adenosine deaminase (ADA) deficiency as tested for by the New York State Newborn Screening Program, some infants were identified who had deficiency of the enzyme in their blood spots but did not have the immunodeficiency that occurs with this disorder. This was explained on the basis of an unstable enzyme in red blood cells that could not be replaced in the absence of a nucleus in these cells.[96] Lymphocytes could compensate for the unstable enzyme by producing new enzyme. Instability of two other enzymes, glutathione reductase[97] and glucose-6-phosphate dehydrogenase,[98] results in hemolytic anemia, but rarely in other systemic effects, because the enzyme deficiency is confined to red blood cells.

Mutations may also increase the stability of proteins, resulting in decreased turnover. Mutations causing increased stability of thyroxine-binding prealbumin *(transthyretin)* result in this protein being deposited in tissues rather than being destroyed, thereby producing disease. These mutations have been shown to be associated with familial amyloid polyneuropathy, amyloidosis, and amyloid cardiomyopathy.[99,100]

GENETIC SUSCEPTIBILITY TO DISEASE

Genes can alter an individual's susceptibility to disease. The susceptibility to disease can be intrinsic to the genetic alteration. In inborn errors of metabolism, the depletion of enzymatic activity results in the accumulation of substrate that itself may be toxic (e.g., sphingolipids in lysosomal storage diseases),[101] or the substrate may be metabolized through another pathway into a toxic substance (e.g., androgens in congenital adrenal hyperplasia).[102] An insufficient amount of gene product may have an adverse effect on subsequent steps in a cascade (e.g., factor VIII clotting factor disorders),[103] or the altered product may accumulate and itself be toxic (transthyretin in amyloidosis).

Alternatively, the genetic alteration may increase susceptibility to external factors causing disease. In individuals who carry a defect in their pro-α (I) collagen genes resulting in osteogenesis imperfecta, the susceptibility to fractures has been increased. These patients develop fractures in response to minimal physical trauma. The susceptibility to genetic disease may be altered by environmental manipulation. In inborn errors of metabolism associated with substrate accumulation, dietary restriction of the offending substance may mitigate or eliminate the disease phenotype.[104] Residual activity of the deficient enzyme may be enhanced by treatment with large amounts of vitamin cofactors.[105] Alternative metabolic pathways may be created through the use of drugs, for example, waste nitrogen in hyperammonic states can be excreted as hippuric acid through the use of sodium benzoate.[7]

The time course with which disease develops depends on the severity of the genetic defect and the ability of alternative pathways to balance or offset the effects of the genetic defect. As a result, the spectrum of disease can be quite variable for individuals who have inherited comparable mutations.

For many genetic conditions, variability in the age of onset and the severity of disease are the rule rather than the exception. The variability is observed even for siblings who share apparently identical environments. This observation suggests that factors in addition to the activities of a single mutant gene and the physical environment in which it operates produce human variability.

REFERENCES

1. Watson JD, Crick FHC. Molecular structure of nucleic acids. Nature 171:737, 1953.
2. Schmid CW, Deininger PL. Sequence organization of the human genome. Cell 6:345–358, 1975.
3. Saunders GF, Chuang CR, Sawada H. Genome complexity and in vivo transcription in human leukemic leukocytes. Acta Haematol 54:227–233, 1975.
4. Berezney R, Coffey DS. The nuclear protein matrix: isolation, structure, and functions. Adv Enzyme Regul 14:63–100, 1976.
5. Adolphs KW, Cheng SM, Paulson JR, Laemmli UK. Isolation of a protein scaffold from mitotic HeLa cell chromosomes. Proc Natl Acad Sci USA 74:4937–4941, 1977.

6. Cheng JF, Smith CL, Cantor CR. Isolation and characterization of a human telomere. Nucleic Acids Res 17:6109–6127, 1989.

7. Cross SH, Allshire RC, McKay SJ, McGill NI, Cooke HJ. Cloning of human telomeres by complementation in yeast. Nature 338:771–774, 1989.

8. Doolittle WF, Sapienza C. Selfish genes, the phenotype paradigm and genome evolution. Nature 284:601–603, 1980.

9. Hickey DA. Selfish DNA: a sexually-transmitted nuclear parasite. Genetics 101:519–531, 1982.

10. Cavalier-Smith T. Selfish DNA and the origin of introns. Nature 315:293–294, 1985.

11. Hwu HR, Roberts JW, Davidson EH, Britten RJ. Insertion and/or deletion of many repeated DNA sequences in human and higher ape evolution. Proc Natl Acad Sci USA 83:3875–3879, 1980.

12. Tashima M, Calabretta B, Torelli G, Scofield M, Maizel A, Saunders GF. Presence of a highly repetitive and widely dispersed DNA sequence in the human genome. Proc Natl Acad Sci USA 78:1508–1512, 1981.

13. Jelinek WR, Schmid CW. Repetitive sequences in eukaryotic DNA and their expression. Annu Rev Biochem 51:813, 1982.

14. Schmickel RD, Knoller M. Characterization and localization of the human genes for ribosomal ribonucleic acid. Pediatr Res 11:929–935, 1977.

15. Carozzi N, Masachi F, Plumb M, Zimmerman S, Zimmerman A, Coles LS, et al. Clustering of human H1 and core histone genes. Science 224:1115–1117, 1984.

16. Orkin SH. The duplicated human alpha globins lie close together in cellular DNA. Proc Natl Acad Sci USA 75:5950–5954, 1978.

17. Chu ML, Myers JC, Bernard MP, Ding JF, Ramirez F. Cloning and characterization of five overlapping cDNAs specific for the human pro alpha. Nucleic Acids Res 10:5925–5934, 1982.

18. Fuchs E, Marchuk D. Type I and Type II keratins have evolved from lower eukaryotes to form the epidermal intermediate filaments in mammlian skin. Proc Natl Acad Sci USA 80:5857–5861, 1983.

19. Fuchs EV, Coppock SM, Green H, Cleveland DW. Two distinct classes of keratin genes and their evolutionary significance. Cell 27:75–84, 1981.

20. Gonzalez IL, Sylvester JE, Smith TF, Stambolian D, Schmickel RD. Ribosomal RNA gene sequences and hominoid phylogeny. Mol Biol Evol 7:203–219, 1990.

21. Stein GS, Stein JL, van Wijnen AJ, Lian JB. Regulation gene expression. Curr Opin Cell Biol 4:166–173, 1992.

22. Fiddes JC, Seeburg PH, DeNoto FM, Hallewell RA, Baxter JD, Goodman HM. Structure of genes for human growth hormone and chorionic somatomammotropin. Proc Natl Acad Sci USA 76:4294–4298, 1979.

23. Seeburg PH. The human growth hormone family: nucleotide sequences show recent divergence and predict a new polypeptide hormone. DNA 1:239–249, 1982.

24. Barsh GS, Seeburg PH, Gelinas RE. The human growth hormone gene family: structure and evolution of the chromosomal locus. Nucleic Acids Res 11:3939–3958, 1983.

25. Strange PG. Receptors for neurotransmitters and related substances. Curr Opin Biotechnol 2:269–277, 1991.

26. Lameh J, Cone RI, Maeda S, Philip M, Corbani M, Nadasdi L, et al. Structure and function of G protein coupled receptors. Pharm Res 7:1213–1221, 1990.

27. Fryxell KJ. The evolutionary divergence of neurotransmitter receptors and second-messenger pathways. J Mol Evol 41:85–97, 1995.

28. Honjo T, Habu S. Origin of immune diversity: genetic variation and selection. Annu Rev Biochem 54:803–830, 1985.

29. Hood L, Kronenberg M, Hunkapiller T. T cell antigen receptors and the immunoglobulin supergene family. Cell 40:225–229, 1985.

30. Ruoslahti E, Terry WD. Alpha fetoprotein and serum albumin show sequence homology. Nature 260:804–805, 1976.

31. Crick FH. The genetic code—yesterday, today, and tomorrow. Cold Spring Harb Symp Quant Biol 31:1–9, 1966.

32. Mathews MB. Mammalian messenger RNA. Essays Biochem 9:59–102, 1973.

33. Jacob ST. Mammalian RNA polymerases. Prog Nucleic Acid Res Mol Biol 13:93–126, 1973.

34. Chamberlin MJ. The selectivity of transcription. Annu Rev Biochem 43:721–775, 1974.

35. Wilt FH. Polyadenylation of maternal RNA of sea urchin eggs after fertilization. Proc Natl Acad Sci USA 70:2345–2349, 1973.

36. Berk AJ, Sharp PA. Spliced early mRNAs of simian virus 40. Proc Natl Acad Sci USA 75:1274–1278, 1978.

37. Wei CM, Moss B. Methylated nucleotides block 5'-terminus of vaccinia virus messenger RNA. Proc Natl Acad Sci USA 72:318–322, 1975.

38. Wei CM, Gershowitz A, Moss B. Methylated nucleotides block 5' terminus of HeLa cell messenger RNA. Cell 4:379–386, 1975.

39. Chen BP, Pestka S. Studies on the formation of transfer ribonucleic acid-ribosome complexes. XIV. Preparation of ribosomes from human placenta: characteristics and requirements of aminoacyl-tRNA binding. Arch Biochem Biophys 148:161–168, 1972.

40. Sundharadas G, Katz JR, Soll D, Konigsberg W, Lengyel P. On the recognition of serine transfer RNAs specific for unrelated codons by the same seryl-transfer RNA synthetase. Proc Natl Acad Sci USA 61:693–700, 1968.

41. Gallo RC, Pestka S. Transfer RNA species in normal and leukemic human lymphoblasts. J Mol Biol 52:195–219, 1970.

42. Skoultchi A, Ono Y, Waterson J, Lengyel P. Peptide chain elongation; indications for the binding of an amino acid polymerization factor, guanosine 5'-triphosphate-aminoacyl transfer ribonucleic acid complex to the messenger-ribosome complex. Biochem 9:508–514, 1970.

43. Ono Y, Skoultchi A, Waterson J, Lengyel P. Peptide chain elongation: GTP cleavage catalysed by factors binding aminoacyl-transfer RNA to the ribosome. Nature 222:645–648, 1969.

44. Ono Y, Skoultchi A, Waterson J, Lengyel P. Stoichiometry of aminoacyl-transfer RNA binding and GTP cleavage during chain elongation and translocation. Nature 223:697–701, 1969.

45. Weiner AM, Weber K. A single UGA codon functions as a natural termination signal in the coliphage q beta coat protein cistron. J Mol Biol 80:837–855, 1973.

46. Paynton C, Sarkar G, Sommer SS. Identification of mutations in two families with sporadic hemophilia A. Hum Genet 87:397–400, 1991.

47. Model P, Webster RE, Zinder ND. The UGA codon in vitro: chain termination and suppression. J Mol Biol 43:177–190, 1969.

48. Beaudet AL, Caskey CT. Mammalian peptide chain termination. II. Codon specificity and GTPase activity of release factor. Proc Natl Acad Sci USA 68:619–624, 1971.

49. Last JA, Stanley WM, Jr., Salas M, Hille MB, Wahba AJ, Ochoa S. Translation of the genetic message. IV. UAA as a chain termination codon. Proc Natl Acad Sci USA 57:1062–1067, 1967.

50. Burke DC. Processing of alphavirus-specific proteins in infected cells. Med Biol 53:352–356, 1975.

51. Blobel G, Dobberstein B. Transfer to proteins across membranes. II. Reconstitution of functional rough microsomes from heterologous components. J Cell Biol 67:852–862, 1975.

52. Blobel G, Dobberstein B. Transfer of proteins across membranes. I. Presence of proteolytically processed and unprocessed nascent immunoglobulin light chains on membrane-bound ribosomes of murine myeloma. J Cell Biol 67:835–851, 1975.

53. van den Berg J, van Ooyen A, Mantei N, Schambock A, Grosveld G, Flavell RA, et al. Comparison of cloned rabbit and mouse beta-globin genes showing strong evolutionary divergence of two homologous pairs of introns. Nature 276:37–44, 1978.

54. Nei M, Stephens JC, Saitou N. Methods for computing the standard errors of branching points in an evolutionary tree and their application to molecular data from humans and apes. Mol Biol Evol 2:66–85, 1985.

55. Kimura M. A simple method for estimating evolutionary rates of base substitutions through comparative studies of nucleotide sequences. J Mol Evol 16:111–120, 1980.

56. Matteson KJ, Ostrer H, Chakravarti A, Buetow KH, O'Brien WE, Beaudet AL, et al. A study of restriction fragment length polymorphisms at the human alpha-1-antitrypsin locus. Hum Genet 69:263–267, 1985.

57. Koeberl DD, Bottema CD, Buerstedde JM, Sommer SS. Functionally important regions of the factor IX gene have a low rate of polymorphism and a high rate of mutation in the dinucleotide CpG. Am J Hum Genet 45:448–457, 1989.

58. Watkins DI, Chen ZW, Hughes AL, Hodi FS, Letvin NL. Genetically distinct cell populations in naturally occurring bone marrow—chimeric primates express similar MHC class I gene products. J Immunol 144:3726–3735, 1990.

59. Boyer SH, Scott AF, Kunkel LM, Smith KD. The proportion of all point mutations which are unacceptable: an estimate based on hemoglobin amino acid and nucleotide sequences. Can J Genet Cytol 20:111–137, 1978.

60. Tykocinski ML, Max EE. CG dinucleotide clusters in MHC genes and in 5' demethylated genes. Nucleic Acids Res 12:4385–4396, 1984.

61. Youssoufian H, Kazazian HH, Jr, Phillips DG, Aronis S, Tsiftis G, Brown VA, et al. Recurrent mutations in haemophelia A give evidence for CpG mutation hotspots. Nature 324:380–382, 1986.

62. Bottema CD, Bottema MJ, Ketterling RP, Yoon HS, Janco RL, Phillips JA, III, et al. Why does the human factor IX gene have a G + C content of 40%? Am J Hum Genet 49:839–850, 1991.

63. Kan YW, Dozy AM, Varmus HE, Taylor JM, Holland JP, Lie-Injo LE, et al. Deletion of α-globin genes in haemoglobin-H disease demonstrates multiple alpha-globin structural loci. Nature 255:255–256, 1975.

64. Ottolenghi S, Lanyon WG, Paul J, Williamson R, Weatherall DJ, Clegg JB, et al. The severe form of alpha thalassaemia is caused by a haemoglobin gene deletion. Nature 251:389–392, 1974.

65. Hobbs HH, Russell DW, Brown MS, Goldstein JL. The LDL receptor locus in familial hypercholesterolemia: mutational analysis of a membrane protein. Annu Rev Genet 24:133–170, 1990.

66. Baglioni C. The fusion of two peptide chains in hemoglobin Lepore and its interpretation as a genetic deletion. Proc Natl Acad Sci USA 48:1880–1886, 1962.

67. Kremer EJ, Pritchard M, Lynch M, Yu S, Holman K, Baker E, et al. Mapping of DNA instability at the fragile X to a trinucleotide repeat sequence p(CCG)n. Science 252:1711–1714, 1991.

68. Blank C. Apert's syndrome (a type of acrocephalosyndactyly): observations on a British series of 39 cases. Ann Hum Genet 24:151–164, 1960.

69. Murdoch J, Walker BA, McKusick VA. Parental age effects on the occurrence of new mutations for the Marfan syndrome. Ann Hum Genet 35:331–336, 1972.

70. Herrmann J. Der Einfluss des Zeugungsalters auf die Mutation zu Hamophilie A. Hum Genet 3:1–16, 1966.

71. Chen SH, Zhang M, Lovrien EW, Scott CR, Thompson AR. CG dinucleotide transitions in the factor IX gene account for about half of the point mutations in hemophilia B patients: a Seattle series. Hum Genet 87:177–182, 1991.

72. Rossiter JP, Young M, Kimberland ML, Hutter P, Ketterling RP, Gitschier J, et al. Factor VIII gene inversions causing severe hemophilia A originate almost exclusively in male germ cells. Hum Mol Genet 3:1035–1039, 1994.

73. Nelson K, Holmes LB. Malformations due to presumed spontaneous mutations in newborn infants. N Engl J Med 320:19–23, 1989.

74. Chakravarti A, Buetow KH, Antonarakis SE, Waber PG, Boehm CD, Kazazian HH. Nonuniform recombination within the human beta-globin gene cluster. Am J Hum Genet 36:1239–1258, 1984.

75. Chakravarti A, Phillips JA, III, Mellits KH, Buetow KH, Seeburg PH. Patterns of polymorphism and linkage disequilibrium suggest independent origins of the human growth hormone gene cluster. Proc Natl Acad Sci USA 81:6085–6089, 1984.

76. Risch N, de Leon D, Ozelius L, Kramer P, Almasy L, Singer B, et al. Genetic analysis of idiopathic torsion dystonia in Ashkenazi Jews and their recent descent from a small founder population. Nat Genet 9:152–159, 1995.

77. Hastbacka J, de la Chapelle A, Kaitila I, Sistonen P, Weaver A, Lander E. Linkage disequilibrium mapping in isolated founder populations: diastrophic dysplasia in Finland. Nat Genet 2:204–211, 1992.

78. Sirugo G, Keats B, Fujita R, Duclos F, Purohit K, Koenig M, et al. Friedreich ataxia in Louisiana Acadians: demonstration of a founder effect by analysis of microsatellite-generated extended haplotypes. Am J Hum Genet 50:559–566, 1992.

79. Antonarakis SE, Boehm CD, Serjeant GR, Theisen CE, Dover GJ, Kazazian HH, Jr. Origin of the beta s-globin gene in blacks: the contribution of recurrent mutation or gene conversion or both. Proc Natl Acad Sci USA 81:853–856, 1984.

80. Eisensmith RC, Okano Y, Dasovich M, Wang T, Guttler F, Lou H, et al. Multiple origins for phenylketonuria in Europe. Am J Hum Genet 51:1355–1365, 1992.

81. Kazazian HH, Jr., Gender GD, Snyder PG, VanBeneden RJ, Woodhead AP. Further evidence of a quantitative deficiency of chain-specific globin mRNA in the thalassemia syndromes. Proc Natl Acad Sci USA 72:567–571, 1975.

82. Perutz MF, Pulsinelli P, Eyck LT, Kilmartin JV, Shibata S, Miyaji Y, et al. Haemoglobin Hiroshima and the mechanism of the alkaline Bohr effect. Nature 232:147–149, 1971.

83. Hamilton HB, Iuchi I, Miyaji T, Shibata S. Hemoglobin Hiroshima (beta 143 histidine to aspartic acid): a newly identified fast moving beta chain variant associated with increased oxygen affinity and compensatory erythremia. J Clin Invest 48:525–535, 1969.

84. Reissmann KR, Ruth WE, Nomura T. A human hemoglobin with lowered oxygen affinity and impaired heme-heme interactions. J Clin Invest 40:1826–1833, 1961.

85. Bonaventura J, Riggs A. Hemoglobin Kansas, a human hemoglobin with a neutral amino acid substitution and an abnormal oxygen equilibrium. J Biol Chem 243:980–991, 1968.

86. Wilkins L. The Diagnosis and Treatment of Endocrine Disorders in Childhood and Adolescence. 2nd ed. Springfield, IL: Carles C. Thomas, 1957.

87. Berta P, Hawkins JR, Sinclair AH, Taylor A, Griffiths BL, Goodfellow PN, et al. Genetic evidence equating SRY and the testis-determining factor. Nature 348:448–450, 1990.

88. Pontiggia A, Rimini R, Harley V, Goodfellow PN, Lovell-Badge R, Bianchi ME. Sex reversing mutations affect the architecture of SRY-DNA complexes. EMBO J 13:6115–6124, 1994.

89. Neitz M, Neitz J, Jacobs GH. Spectral tuning of pigments underlying red-green color vision. Science 252:971–974, 1991.

90. Merbs SL, Nathans J. Absorption spectra of the hybrid pigments responsible for anomalous color vision. Science 258:464–466, 1992.

91. Lane EB. Keratin diseases. Curr Opin Genet Dev 4:412–418, 1994.

92. Prockop DJ, Kivirikko KI. Collagens: molecular biology, diseases, and potentials for therapy. Annu Rev Biochem 64:403–434, 1995.

93. Ingram VM. A specific chemical difference between the globins of normal human and sickle cell anemia hemoglobin. Nature 178:792, 1956.

94. Monplaisir N, Merault G, Poyart C, Rhoda MD, Craescu C, Vidaud M, et al. Hemoglobin S Antilles: a variant with lower solubility than hemoglobin S and producing sickle cell disease in heterozygotes. Proc Natl Acad Sci USA 83:9363–9367, 1986.

95. Owen MC, Brennan SO, Lewis JH, Carrell RW. Mutation of antitrypsin to antithrombin. Alpha 1-antitrypsin Pittsburgh (358 Met leads to Arg), a fatal bleeding disorder. New Engl J Med 309:694–698, 1983.

96. Hirschhorn R, Roegner V, Jenkins T, Seaman C, Piomelli S, Borkowsky W. Erythrocyte adenosine deaminase deficiency without immunodeficiency: evidence for an unstable mutant enzyme. J Clin Invest 64:1130–1139, 1979.

97. Lohr GW, Waller HD. Eine neue enzymopenische haemolytische Anaemie mit Glutathionreduktase-Mangel. Med Klin 57:1521–1525, 1962.

98. Beutler E, Mathai CK, Smith JE. Biochemical variants of glucose-6-phosphate dehydrogenase giving rise to congenital nonspherocytic hemolytic disease. Blood 31:131–150, 1968.

99. Costa PP, Figueira AS, Bravo FR. Amyloid fibril protein related to prealbumin in familial amyloidotic polyneuropathy. Proc Natl Acad Sci USA 75:4499–4503, 1978.

100. Koeppen AH, Mitzen EJ, Hans MB, Peng SK, Bailey RO. Familial amyroid polyneuropathy. Muscle Nerve 8:733–749, 1985.

101. Okada S, O'Brien JS. Tay-Sachs disease: generalized absence of a beta-D-N-acetylhexosaminidase component. Science 165:698–700, 1969.

102. Bongiovanni AM, Root AW. The adrenogenital syndrome. New Engl J Med 268:1283, 1342, 1391–1289, 1351, 1399, 1963.

103. Rapaport SI, Patch MJ, Moore FJ. Anti-hemophilic globulin levels in carriers of hemophilia. J Clin Invest 39:1619–1625, 1960.

104. Bickel H, Gerard J, Hickmans EM. The influence of phenylalanine intake on the chemistry and behavior of a phenylketonuric child. Acta Paediatr 43:64–77, 1954.

105. Mudd SH. Vitamin-responsive genetic disease. J Clin Pathol 27:38, 1974.

3

Deviations From
The Mendelian Paradigm

The familial transmission of color blindness in humans demonstrates that Mendel's laws are insufficient to explain the genetics of this condition in humans. Typically, the color-blind individual is born to unaffected parents, and on average, one-quarter of the offspring in these families have the condition. The uninformed observer might conclude that color blindness is a recessive condition based on the ratio of 3:1 for affected to unaffected. Yet the same observer would be hard-pressed to fit a model of autosomal recessive inheritance based on its occurrence only in male offspring and the presence of the same condition in the transmitting mother's brothers and maternal uncles. In some families, hemophilia A is transmitted along with color blindness. When confronted with this problem, Bell and Haldane concluded (correctly) that the genes for the two traits were linked.[1]

In 1657, Sir William Harvey, the discoverer of the circulatory system, stated,

Nature is nowhere accustomed more openly to display her secret mysteries than in cases where she shows traces of her workings apart from the beaten path; nor is there any better way to advance the proper practice of medicine than to give our minds to discovery of the usual laws of nature by careful investigation of cases of rarer forms of disease. For it has been found, in almost all things, that what they contain of useful or applicable is hardly perceived unless we are deprived of them, or they become deranged in some way.

Both color blindness and hemophilia A are the exception rather than the rule in the population. Approximately 5–10% of males worldwide have color blindness, and one in every 5,000 to 10,000 males has hemophilia A.[2] These conditions occur together rarely (one in every 50,000 to 200,000 males). Thus, it was analysis of exceptional cases such as these that demonstrated X-linked transmission and genetic linkage in humans.

Analysis of phenotypes and transmission ratios for many familial conditions have highlighted other exceptions to Mendel's rules. Phenotypes can vary both quantitatively and qualitatively from one individual to another. Quantitative variation means that a condition develops at an earlier age or with greater severity. Quantitative variation may also mean that some individuals who are obligate genetic carriers do not show any phenotypic features of the condition ("nonpenetrance").

The presence of such nonpenetrant individuals may cause apparent deviation from the predicted Mendelian transmission ratio. Deviation from Mendelian transmission ratios also occurs for sporadic genetic conditions in which the affected individuals do not reproduce, and for conditions that demonstrate preferential transmission from either the mother or the father. Each of these deviations from Mendelian transmission is reviewed in this chapter.

VARIABLE EXPRESSIVITY

Variable expressivity is the term that is used to describe the quantitative and qualitative variation in Mendelian phenotypes within a family. When viewed in terms of a Mendelian disorder, the severity may vary among the affected members in a family because (1) some, but not all, features of the disease state are present, (2) the actual severity of any one feature is greater, (3) the age of onset varies, or (4) monozygotic twins are discordant for the condition.

Variation in the features of a complex phenotype. The severity of a Mendelian disorder can vary not only in the degree of disability but also in the specific features that are present. Such variation is observed for many different conditions and can be illustrated be a few examples. Stickler syndrome, or hereditary progressive arthro-ophthalmopathy, is a disorder of connective tissue resulting from alterations in type II or type XI collagen.[3-5] Individuals with Stickler syndrome are affected variably with myopia, retinal detachment, small chin with cleft palate *(Robin sequence),* deafness, early arthritis, and mitral valve prolapse (Fig. 3.1).[6-10] Several of these features, including retinal detachment, deafness, Robin sequence, and mitral valve prolapse, do not occur consistently among members of a family.

Waardenburg syndrome, type I, is a condition of abnormal pigmentation affecting eyes, ears, skin, and hair that is thought to result from the abnormal migration of pigment-bearing cells.[11-15] Within a family, individuals may vary in their presentation with some having white spots on their skin, a white forelock of hair, different-colored eyes (heterochromia), or some combination thereof. Furthermore, some individuals have sensorineural hearing loss, whereas others do not.

Neurofibromatosis is also a condition of abnormal pigmentation. Characteristic

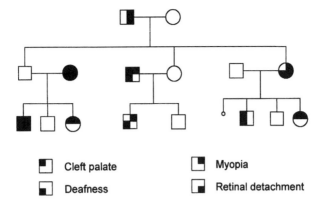

Cleft palate	Myopia
Deafness	Retinal detachment

Figure 3.1. Pedigree of Stickler syndrome demonstrating variable expressivity as the manifestation of different phenotypic features.

brown areas on the body, termed *café-au-lait* spots,[16–18] are present. Affected individuals may develop benign tumors anywhere on their bodies. Within a family, some individuals may have only café-au-lait spots and benign tumors in the pigmented regions of their eyes, termed *Lisch nodules,*[19,20] whereas others develop tumors on their skin or in other locations. About 2% of the time, individuals with neurofibromatosis I develop malignancies, especially neurofibrosarcomas. The absence of malignancies in previous generations does not eliminate the risk of malignancy for an affected individual.

Li-Fraumeni syndrome is a condition in which different tumors may occur among different members of a family.[21,22] Some members have myelogeous leukemia, whereas others develop breast cancer or soft-tissue sarcomas (Fig. 3.2).

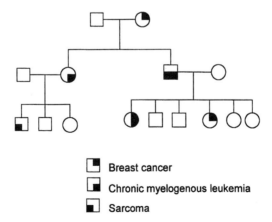

Breast cancer
Chronic myelogenous leukemia
Sarcoma

Figure 3.2. Pedigree of Li-Fraumeni syndrome demonstrating variable expressivity as the occurrence of different tumors.

Sometimes an affected individual may develop more than one kind of cancer. All of these conditions, Stickler syndrome, Waardenburg syndrome, neurofibromatosis I, and Li-Fraumeni syndrome, reveal variation in the features of a complex phenotype—examples of variable expressivity.

Variation in disease severity. When the actual severity of any one feature is greater compared to other affected family members, there may be more frequent illness, greater disability, or earlier death compared to other family members. Some children with the brittle bone disease osteogenesis imperfecta are born with fractures and deforming skeletal abnormalities. By contrast, their parents may develop fractures later in life, and only in response to trauma.[23–25]

Likewise, the severity of Marfan syndrome, another disorder of connective tissue, can be variable. Affected individuals usually have myopia, dislocated lenses, scoliosis, hyperextensible joints, mitral valve prolapse, and aortic root dilatation.[26,27] The aortic dilatation may progress to an aneurysm with dissection. Although aortic aneurysms represent the major cause of mortality in Marfan syndrome, their occurrence is highly variable.

Variation in the age at onset and rate of progression. Both the age at onset and the rate of progression may vary among affected individuals in families with some genetic disorders. Polycystic kidney disease is a progressive autosomal dominant disorder. The first signs of disease are the development of cysts in the kidney that may disrupt blood vessels and lead to the development of blood in the urine. Ordinarily, polycystic kidney disease progresses to end-stage renal failure, requiring dialysis and transplantation. The ages at which cysts and renal failure are observed usually vary from one affected family member to another.[28–32]

Variability in the age at onset, number of symptoms, and the rate of progression is also observed for myotonic dystrophy, a muscle disease associated with muscle weakness, sustained contraction of the muscle *(myotonia)*, cataracts, baldness, and sometimes mental retardation. Unlike some of the conditions discussed above, the age at onset in succeeding generations tends to be earlier (Fig. 3.3).[33,34]

Discordance between monozygotic twins. A special case of variable expressivity is that of monozygotic twins, who would be expected to have the same phenotype, but do not. Several monozygotic twins have been described in which one twin had normal male genitalia and the other had female genitalia (Fig. 3.4).[35–37] Female monozygotic twin pairs with Duchenne muscular dystrophy have been described in which one has profound muscle weakness and rapid progression, whereas the other has minimal weakness, if any.[38,39] In fact, the only sign of disease in the mildly affected twin has been elevation of the concentration of the muscle enzyme creatinine phosphokinase in serum. This elevation indicates that some muscle damage has occurred in the less severely affected twin.

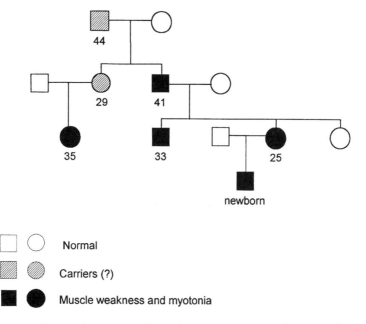

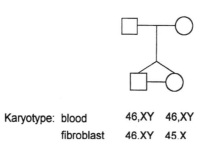

Normal

Carriers (?)

Muscle weakness and myotonia

Figure 3.3. Pedigree of myotonic dystrophy demonstrating earlier age of onset in subsequent generations.

DEVIATION FROM MENDELIAN TRANSMISSION

Deviation from Mendelian transmission ratios may occur by chance alone, especially if the family size is small. Several other explanations have been developed to explain these deviations. They include: (1) nonpenetrant cases, (2) sporadic cases, (3) preferential parental transmission, and (4) multifactorial inheritance.

Nonpenetrant cases. The limiting case of variable expressivity is not manifesting any signs of the disease state. By linkage analysis or direct analysis of the mutation, the nonpenetrant individual can be shown to carry a gene for this

Karyotype: blood   46,XY   46,XY
fibroblast   46.XY   45.X

Figure 3.4. Monozygotic twins discordant for sexual phenotype.

condition. In the fragile X mental retardation syndrome, normal transmitting males have the gene for this condition, but they are not mentally retarded (Fig. 3.5).[40]

The boundary between mild expression and nonpenetrance can be quite subtle. Some parents of children with retinoblastoma, a malignant tumor of childhood, have been unaware that they carried this gene until the birth of an affected child. Subsequent careful examination demonstrated the presence of benign retinomas in their eyes; thus, it is possible for individuals to be penetrant for this condition without their knowledge.[41]

Sporadic cases. Some conditions are genetic, but sporadic, because they occur only once within a family. Although autosomal dominant, autosomal recessive, and X-linked forms of retinitis pigmentosa have all been demonstrated (chapter 2), in up to 50% of cases, the presenting individual is the first case to be identified in the family.[42,43] For such individuals it is not obvious which gene, nor which pattern of inheritance, is associated with his or her disease.

Preferential parental transmission. For some genetic conditions, parents may have a larger number of affected children than would be predicted from inheritance of a single disease allele. Mothers affected with Leber hereditary optic neuropathy have a 60% chance of having affected children. Moreover, transmission of Leber hereditary optic neuropathy occurs only from affected mothers, not from affected fathers (Fig.3.6).[44,45]

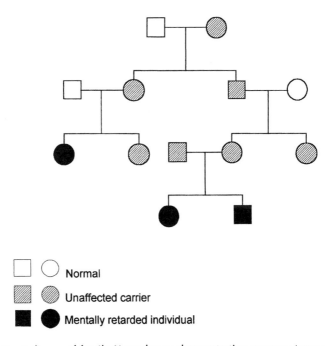

☐ ◯ Normal

▨ ◐ Unaffected carrier

■ ● Mentally retarded individual

Figure 3.5. Pedigree of fragile X syndrome demonstrating nonpenetrance.

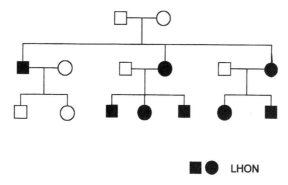

LHON

Figure 3.6. Pedigree with Leber hereditary optic neuropathy demonstrating maternal transmission.

Preferential transmission by the parent of one sex has been observed for other conditions. In familial Beckwith-Wiedeman syndrome (BWS), affected infants are large at birth and have large tongues, abdominal wall openings *(omphaloceles),* and excess insulin secretion, resulting in hypoglycemia. In most familial cases, the condition is transmitted only by mothers—not by fathers.[46–48] Equal numbers of male and female infants are affected and a few cases of father-to-son transmission have been described, suggesting that, unlike color blindness and hemophilia A, the gene for this condition is not X-linked.[47,48]

Multifactorial inheritance. Some conditions that occur within a family are termed *multifactorial* because multiple genes and environmental effects are thought to contribute to the development of the phenotype. One indication of multifactorial inheritance is the observation that the number of affected individuals in a family cannot be predicted from inheritance of a single gene, including one with reduced penetrance. Cleft lip may occur with or without an associated cleft palate, and the inheritance is multifactorial. Among the first-, second-, and third-degree relatives of an affected individual, the risks of cleft lip with or without cleft palate are 4%, 0.7%, and 0.3%.[49] These risks fall off more rapidly than would be predicted from transmission of a single gene of low penetrance.

Ascertainment or typing errors. Some apparent violations of Mendelian inheritance can be explained in genetic terms without revoking the paradigm (Table 3.1). Incomplete ascertainment or typing errors result when affected individuals are misclassified as unaffected (or the opposite). Such errors are more likely to occur when typing is performed on the basis of history, rather than direct observation, or where there have been multiple observers performing typing by different criteria.

The distribution of a quantitative phenotype may be very broad, so the same individual may have very different values if sampled at different times. For example, both plasma amino acid and circulating hormone concentrations show significant variation that may be influenced by diet or time of day.[50–53] Precise

Table 3.1. Some Ways to Explain Deviations from the Mendelian Paradigm

Ascertainment errors
Parental reproductive choice
Decreased reproductive fitness
Stochastic variation
Modifying genes

phenotypic analysis may require control of the environmental variation by sampling at different times of the day or in response to a dietary load of substrate.

Parental reproductive choice. Parental reproductive choice can alter the ratio of affected to unaffected. For some genetic disorders, parents choose to have small families or they may choose not to have any additional children once a child has been born with a severe condition. Methods of pedigree analysis have been developed to account for these sources of bias.[54]

Decreased reproductive fitness. For some conditions, the reproductive fitness is markedly decreased because of early lethality, abnormalities of the reproductive system, or profound mental retardation; thus, the likelihood that affected individuals will have offspring is low. As a result, there may be too few cases to be confident of a genetic pattern of transmission. Although there may be a genetic basis for such sporadic cases, it can only be demonstrated by association with a specific genetic marker.

Modifying genes. Modifying genes represent another cause of variation. The concept of modifying genes is almost as old as the field of human genetics itself. In the 1920s, R. A. Fisher proposed that modifying genes are polymorphic.[55–57] The phenotype depends on which of the alleles is inherited. In eukaryotic organisms other than humans, the effect of a modifying gene became known as *epistasis*. In these organisms, it was possible to test whether one locus was epistatic to another through a series of genetic crosses which tested whether the expression of the alleles at one locus was modified by the alleles at a second.

Evidence for modifying genes in humans has been harder to come by. One of the first examples was for sickle cell disease. Milder disease was observed in individuals within certain families or ethnic groups who had elevated fetal hemoglobin concentrations. The severity of the disease varied inversely with the fetal hemoglobin concentration, so individuals who were homozygous for the sickle cell mutation and had fetal hemoglobin concentrations of 20% or greater did not have any disease at all.[58,59]

Hereditary persistence of fetal hemoglobin (HPFH) is an accentuation of the process of incomplete switching from fetal to adult hemoglobin synthesis that takes place around the time of birth. On a cellular level, HPFH has been demonstrated to occur either in all red blood cells (pancellular) or only in a fraction of red blood cells (heterocellular). Gamma globin is synthesized from each of two different genes, termed $^A\gamma$ and $^G\gamma$. As a result, two forms of pancellular HPFH have been observed.[60] In one form, there is increased production of $^A\gamma$ subunits,[61,62] whereas in the other form there is increased production of $^G\gamma$.[63] Each form of pancellular HPFH is inherited as an autosomal dominant trait. Mutations in the regulatory regions of the $^A\gamma$ and $^G\gamma$ genes lead to increased production of the gene product; thus, the γ-globin loci can be modifiers of the phenotype produced by the S allele at the β-globin locus.

A completely different set of modifiers causes the heterocellular form of HPFH. Linkage analysis has demonstrated that the modifying loci map to the β-globin gene complex on chromosome 11,[64] to the X chromosome,[65] or elsewhere.[66] These modifiers are presumed to operate by regulating γ-globin gene expression, although their specific mechanisms are unknown.

Hereditary persistence of fetal hemoglobin is representative of the class of genetic modifiers in which one product substitutes for another and mitigates the effect of that deleterious product. These modifiers may act directly (i.e., pancellular HPFH) or as part of a regulatory cascade (i.e., heterocellular HPFH). Modifying genes may also work by altering a gene product.

The ABO blood groups represent an example of modification of a gene product.[67] The A and B blood groups result from glycosylation of the H antigen gene product.[8] The O blood group results from absence of A or B.[68] There are two ways that this can occur; either from failure to express the H antigen (also known as the Bombay blood group)[69] or from failure to glycosylate the H antigen as the result of mutation in the gene for the glycosyltransferase.[70]

Deviation from the Mendelian paradigm not explained by Mendelian models. Deviations from the Mendelian paradigm are not resolved in all cases by the observations discussed above. Other genetic models have been developed to explain some of the observed deviations. The validity of these models has been tested using the available genetic markers. In some instances, the process has worked in reverse: Observations have been made about aberrant transmission of genetic markers; then theory was developed (or revisited) to explain the observations.

In the next series of chapters in this book, processes that were not foreseen by Mendel and his intellectual heirs are reviewed. These processes are not explained by the stable transmission of polymorphic linked genes on human chromosomes in germ cells. Rather these deviations from the Mendelian paradigm reflect aberrant transmission from human chromosomes that are the result of errors in meiosis or mitosis, of chromosomal rearrangement, or of chromosomal instability. Some of these deviations reflect the unequal contributions of the maternal and paternal genome, high rates of new mutation in the genomes of germ or somatic cells, and the distribution of cells bearing new mutations, resulting in genetic mosaicism. In addition, some of these deviations reflect the contributions of the mitochondrial genome and of exogenous genetic elements.

REFERENCES

1. Bell J, Haldane JBS. The linkage between the genes for color-blindness and haemophilia in men. Proc R Soc Lond [Biol]123:119–150, 1937.
2. Hurvich LM. Color Vision. Sunderland: Sinauer, 1981.
3. Francomano CA, Liberfarb RM, Hirose T, Maumenee IH, Streeten EA, Meyers DA, et al. The Stickler syndrome: evidence for close linkage to the structural gene for type II collagen. Genomics 4:293–296, 1987.
4. Brunner HG, van Beersum SEC, Warman ML, Olsen BR, Ropers H-H, Mariman ECM. A Stickler syndrome gene is linked to chromosome 6 near the COL11A2 gene. Hum Mol Genet 3:1561–1564, 1994.
5. Vikkula M, Mariman ECM, Lui VCH, Zhidkova NI, Tiller GE, Goldring MB, et al. Autosomal dominant and recessive osteochondrodysplasias associated with the COL11A2 locus. Cell 80:431–437, 1995.
6. Hall J. Stickler syndrome presenting as a syndrome of cleft palate, myopia and blindness inherited as a dominant trait. Birth Defects 10:157–171, 1974.
7. Herman J, France TD, Spanger JW, Opitz JM, Wiffler C. The Stickler syndrome (hereditary arthroophthalmopathy). Birth Defects 11:76–103, 1975.
8. Stickler GB, Belau PG, Farrell FJ, Jones JD, Pugh DG, Steinberg AG, et al. Hereditary progressive arthro-ophthalmopathy. Mayo Clin Proc 40:433–455, 1965.
9. Blair NP, Albert DM, Liberfarb RM, Hirose T. Hereditary progressive arthro-ophthalmopathy of Stickler. Am J Ophthalmol 88:876–888, 1979.
10. Liberfarb RM, Hirose T, Holmes LB. The Wagner-Stickler syndrome: a study of 22 families. J Pediatr 99:394–399, 1981.
11. Arias S. Genetic heterogeneity in the Waardenburg syndrome. Birth Defects 7:87–101, 1971.
12. Houghton NI. Waardenberg's syndrome with deafness as the presenting symptom: report or two cases. N Z Med J 63:83–89, 1964.
13. Pantke OA, Cohen MM, Jr. The Waardenberg syndrome. Birth Defects 7:147–152, 1971.
14. da-Silva EO. Waardenburg I syndrome: a clinical and genetic study of two large Brazilian kindreds, and literature review. Am J Hum Genet 40:65–74, 1991.
15. Preus M, Linstrom C, Polomeno RC, Milot J. Waardenburg syndrome: penetrance of major signs. Am J Hum Genet 15:383–388, 1983.
16. Riccardi VM. Von Recklinghausen neurofibromatosis. N Engl J Med 305:1617–1626, 1981.
17. Riccardi VM, Eichner JE. Neurofibromatosis: Phenotype, Natural History and Pathogenesis. Baltimore: Johns Hopkins University Press, 1986.
18. Philippart M. Neurofibromatose hereditaire a large spectre phenotypique (famille SN). J Genet Hum 10:338–346, 1961.
19. Lisch K. Ueber Beteiligung der Augen, insbesonders das Vorkommen von Irisknotchen bei der Neurofibromatose (Recklinghausen). Augenheilkunde 93:137–143, 1937.
20. Zehavi C, Romano A, Goodman RM. Iris (Lisch) nodules in neurofibromatosis. Clin Genet 29:51–55, 1986.
21. Li FP, Fraumeni JF. Soft-tissue sarcomas, breast cancer, and other neoplasms: a familial syndrome? Ann Intern Med 71:747–752, 1969.
22. Lynch HT, Mulcahy GM, Harris RE, Guirgis HA, Lynch JF. Genetic and pathologic findings in a kindred with hereditary sarcoma breast cancer, brain tumors,

leukemia, lung, laryngeal, and adrenal cortical carcinoma. Cancer 41:2055–2064, 1978.

23. Wallis GA, Starman BJ, Zinn AB, Byers PH. Variable expression of osteogenesis imperfecta in a nuclear family is explained by somatic mosaicism for a lethal point mutation in the alpha 1(I) gene (COL1A1) of type I collagen in a parent. Am J Hum Genet 46:1034–1040, 1990.

24. Constantinou CD, Pack M, Young SB, Prockop DJ. Phenotypic heterogeneity in osteogenesis imperfecta: the mildly affected mother of a proband with a lethal variant has the same mutation substituting cysteine for alpha 1-glycine 904 in a type I procollagen gene (COL1A1). Am J Hum Genet 47:670–679, 1990.

25. Mottes M, Sangalli A, Valli M, Gomez Lira M, Tenni R, Buttitta P, et al. Mild dominant osteogenesis imperfecta with intrafamilial variability: the cause is a serine for glycine alpha 1(I) 901 substitution in a type-I collagen gene. Hum Genet 89:480–484, 1992.

26. McKusick VA. The cardiovascular aspect of Marfan's syndrome. Circulation 11:321–342, 1955.

27. Pyeritz RE, McKusick VA. The Marfan syndrome. New Engl J Med 300:772–777, 1979.

28. Gal A, Wirth B, Kaarriainen H, Lucotte G, Landais P, Gillessen-Kaesbach G, et al. Childhood manifestation of autosomal dominant polycystic kidney disease: no evidence for genetic heterogeneity. Clin Genet 35:13–19, 1989.

29. Shokeir MHK. Expression of "adult" polycystic renal disease in the fetus and newborn. Clin Genet 14:61–72, 1978.

30. Zerres K, Rudnik-Schoneborn S, Deget F, Beetz R, Brodehl J, Kuwertz-Broking E, et al. Childhood onset autosomal dominant polycystic kidney disease in sibs: clinical picture and recurrence risk. J Med Genet 30:583–588, 1993.

31. Ravine D, Walker RG, Gibson RN, Sheffield LJ, Kincaid-Smith P, Danks DM. Treatable complications in undiagnosed cases of autosomal dominant polycystic kidney disease. Lancet 337:127–129, 1991.

32. Coto E, Aguado S, Alvarez J, Menendez Diaz MJ, Lopez-Larrea C. Genetic and clinical studies in autosomal dominant polycystic kidney disease type 1 (ADPLS1). J Med Genet 29:243–246, 1996.

33. Bell J. On the age of onset and age at death in hereditary muscular dystrophy with some observations bearing on the question of antedating. Ann Eugenics 11:272–289, 1942.

34. Harper PS. Myotonic Dystrophy. Philadelphia: WB Saunders, 1989.

35. Reindollar RH, Byrd JR, Hahn DH, Haseltine FP, McDonough PG. A cytogenetic and endocrinologic study of a set of monozygotic isokaryotic 45,X/46,XY twins discordant for phenotypic sex: mosaicism versus chimerism. Fertil Steril 47:626–633, 1987.

36. Gonsoulin W, Copeland KL, Carpenter RJ, Jr., Hughes MR, Elder FF. Fetal blood sampling demonstrating chimerism in monozygotic twins discordant for sex and tissue karyotype (46,XY and 45,X). Prenat Diagn 10:25–28, 1990.

37. Fujimoto A, Boelter WD, Sparkes RS, Lin MS, Battersby K. Monozygotic twins of discordant sex both with 45,X/46,X,idic(Y) mosaicism. Am J Med Genet 41:239–245, 1991.

38. Richards CS, Watkins SC, Hoffman EP, Schneider NR, Milsark IW, Katz KS, et al. Skewed X inactivation in a female MZ twin results in Duchenne muscular dystrophy. Am J Hum Genet 46:672–681, 1990.

39. Gomez MR, Engel AG, Dewald G, Peterson HA. Failure of inactivation of Du-

chenne dystrophy X-chromosome in one of female identical twins. Neurology 27:537–541, 1977.

40. Sherman SL, Jacobs PA, Morton NE, Froster-Iskenius U, Howard-Peebles PN, Nielsen KB, et al. Further segregation analysis of the fragile X syndrome with special reference to transmitting males. Hum Genet 69:289–299, 1985.

41. Gallie BL, Ellsworth RM, Abramson DM, Phillips RA. Retinoma: spontaneous regression of retinoblastoma or benign manifestation of the mutation? Br J Cancer 45:513–521, 1982.

42. Fishman GA. Retinitis pigmentosa. Genetic percentages. Arch Ophthalmol 96:822–826, 1978.

43. Bundey S, Crews SJ. A study of retinitis pigmentosa in the city of Birmingham. II Clinical and genetic heterogeneity. J Med Genet 21:421–428, 1984.

44. Erickson RP. Leber's hereditary optic atrophy, a possible example of maternal inheritance. Am J Hum Genet 24:348–349, 1972.

45. Nikoskelainen E, Savontaus M, Wanne OP, Katila MJ, Nummelin KU. Leber's hereditary neuroretinopathy, a maternally inherited disease. Arch Ophthalmol 105:665–671, 1987.

46. Lubinsky M, Herrmann J, Kosseff AL, Opitz JM. Autosomal-dominant sex-dependent transmission of the Wiedemann-Beckwith syndrome. Lancet 1:932, 1974.

47. Ping AJ, Reeve AE, Law DJ, Young MR, Boehnke M, Feinberg AP. Genetic linkage of Beckwith-Wiedemann syndrome to 11p15. Am J Hum Genet 44:720–723, 1989.

48. Moutou C, Junien C, Henry I, Bonaiti Pellie C. Beckwith-Wiedemann syndrome: a demonstration of the mechanisms responsible for the excess of transmitting females. J Med Genet 29:217–220, 1992.

49. Habib Z. Genetic counseling and genetics of cleft lip and cleft palate. (Review). Obstet Gynecol Surv 33:441–447, 1978.

50. Milsom JP, Morgan MY, Sherlock S. Factors affecting plasma amino acid concentrations in control subjects. Metab Clin Exp 28:313–319, 1979.

51. Zimmet PZ, Wall JR, Rome R, Stimmler L, Jarrett RJ. Diurnal variation in glucose tolerance: associated changes in plasma insulin, growth hormone, and non-esterified fatty acids. Br Med J 1:485–488, 1974.

52. Katz FH, Romfh P, Smith JA. Diurnal variation of plasma aldosterone, cortisol and renin activity in supine man. J Clin Endocrinol Metab 40:125–134, 1975.

53. Rose RM, Kreuz LE, Holaday JW, Sulak KJ, Kohnson CE. Diurnal variation of plasma testosterone and cortisol. J Endocrinol 54:177–178, 1972.

54. Leonard CO, Chase GA, Childs B. Genetic counseling: a consumers' view. N Engl J Med 287:433–439, 1972.

55. Fisher RA. The possible modification of the response of the wild type to recurrent mutations. Am Nat 62:115–126, 1928.

56. Fisher RA. Two further notes on the origin of dominance. Am Nat 62:571–574, 1928.

57. Wright S. Fisher's theory of dominance. Am Nat 63:274–279, 1929.

58. Huisman TH, Miller A, Schroeder WA. A G gamma type of the hereditary persistence of fetal hemoglobin with beta chain production in cis. Am J Hum Genet 27:765–777, 1975.

59. Stamatoyannopoulos G, Wood WG, Papayannopoulou T, Nute PE. A new form of hereditary persistence of fetal hemoglobin in blacks and its association with sickle cell trait. Blood 46:683–692, 1975.

60. Huisman TH, Schroeder WA, Dozy AM, Shelton JR, Shelton JB, Boyd EM, et al. Evidence for multiple structural genes for the gamma-chain of human fetal meno-

globin in hereditary persistence of fetal hemoglobin. Ann N Y Acad Sci 165:320–331, 1969.

61. Collins FS, Metherall JE, Yamakawa M, Pan J, Weissman SM, Forget BG. A point mutation in the $^A\gamma$-globin gene promotor in Greek hereditary persistence of fetal haemoglobin. Nature 313:325–326, 1985.

62. Gelinas R, Endlich B, Pfeiffer C, Yagi M, Stamatoyannopoulos G. G to A substitution in the distal CCAAT box of the $^A\gamma$-globin gene in Greek hereditary persistence of fetal haemoglobin. Nature 313:323–325, 1985.

63. Collins FS, Boehm CD, Waber PG, Stoeckert CJ, Jr., Weissman SM, Forget BG, et al. Concordance of a point mutation 5-prime to the $^G\gamma$-globin gene with $^G\gamma$-$\beta(+)$ hereditary persistence of fetal hemoglobin in the black population. Blood 64:1292–1296, 1984.

64. Donald JA, Lammi A, Trent RJ. Hemoglobin F production in heterocellular hereditary persistence of fetal hemoglobin and its linkage to the beta globin gene complex. Hum Genet 80:69–74, 1988.

65. Dover GJ, Smith KD, Chang YC, Purvis S, Mays A, Meyers DA, et al. Fetal hemoglobin levels in sickle cell disease and normal individuals are partially controlled by an X-linked gene located at Xp22.2. Blood 80:816–824, 1992.

66. Thein SL, Sampietro M, Rohde K, Rochette J, Weatherall DJ, Lathrop GM, et al. Detection of a major gene for heterocellular hereditary persistence of fetal hemoglobin after accounting for genetic modifiers. Am J Hum Genet 54:214–228, 1994.

67. Landsteiner K. Zur Kenntnis der antifermentativen, lytischen und agglutinierenden Wirkungen des Blutserums und der Lymphe. Zbl Bakt 27:357–362, 1900.

68. Levine P, Robinson E, Celano M, Briggs O, Falkinburg L. Gene interaction resulting in suppression of blood group substance B. Blood 10:1100–1108, 1955.

69. Kelly RJ, Ernst LK, Larsen RD, Bryant JG, Robinson JS, Lowe JB. Molecular basis for H blood group deficiency in Bombay (Oh) and para-Bombay individuals. Proc Natl Acad Sci USA 91: 5843–5847, 1994.

70. Yamamoto F, Clausen H, White T, Marken J, Hakomori S. Molecular genetic basis of the histo-blood group ABO system. Nature 345:229–233, 1990.

.

4

Chromosomal Transmission

Following linkage and sex-linked transmission, aberrant chromosomal transmission was the next series of mechanisms identified as deviations from Mendel's rules.[1] The first piece of evidence in humans came in 1955: Lejeune observed an extra chromosome 21 in individuals with Down syndrome, a condition with mental retardation, short stature, and a predisposition to congenital heart disease, childhood leukemia, and early onset Alzheimer disease.[2] Lejeune's observation was rapidly followed by the demonstration of altered chromosomal constitutions in Turner syndrome and Klinefelter syndrome. Turner syndrome, a condition with short stature, webbed neck, dysgenetic gonads, and frequently coarctation of the aorta and kidney malformations is associated with the absence of a second X chromosome (45,X).[3] Klinefelter syndrome, a condition of tall stature with small testes and incomplete virilization ("eunuchoid habitus") is associated with the presence of an extra X chromosome (47, XXY).[4] Subsequently, other abnormalities in chromosomal replication, recombination, and transmission were identified.

NORMAL CHROMOSOMAL TRANSMISSION

The transmission of chromosomes from parents to offspring provides the physical basis for Mendelian inheritance.[5] In the gametes (egg and sperm cell precursors—mature germ cells), the chromosomes undergo a series of processes that are collectively known as *meiosis* (Fig. 4.1). These processes include replication of the chromosomes, recombination between the copies *(chromatids)* of each of the homologous chromosomes, and then a series of cell divisions that lead to the presence of one copy of each chromosome in the egg and sperm cells.

Mendelian inheritance also requires that, following fertilization, the chromosomes be faithfully replicated and transmitted from parental to daughter cells.

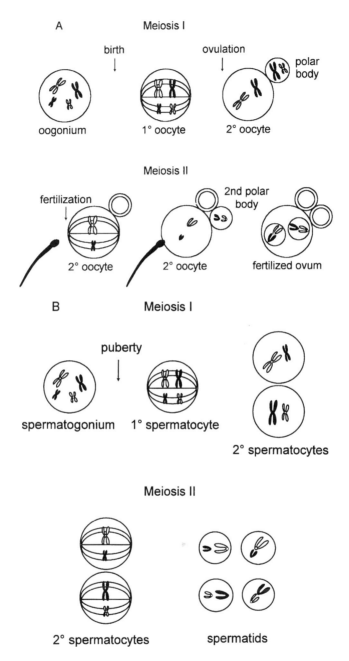

Figure 4.1. Meiosis in female germ cells (A) and in male germ cells (B). The first mitotic division results in a reduction of chromosomes, whereas the second results in a reduction in the number of chromatids.

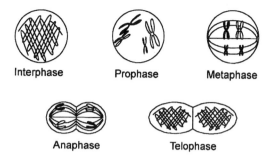

Interphase   Prophase   Metaphase

Anaphase   Telophase

Figure 4.2. Mitosis in somatic cells. The chromosomes replicate, then condense and are partitioned to the two daughter cells by the mitotic spindle.

The processes of replication, pairing of homologous chromosomes, and transmission to offspring are known collectively as *mitosis* (Fig. 4.2). Recombination between the two chromosomes in a pair or between the two chromatids on a chromosome is part of the normal processes of chromosomal transmission in somatic cells.[6]

Errors can occur in any of these processes. When the errors occur in germ cells, the effect is to produce zygotes and subsequently organisms whose somatic cells have altered chromosomal constitutions. The transmission of these novel chromosomes may not follow Mendel's rules. In some instances the transmission may be sporadic. In other instances their recurrence in the offspring may be substantially higher or lower than the expected rate of 50%.

Errors in chromosomal replication and transmission may be confined to somatic cells.[7] As a result the phenotypic effects may occur only in the host and not be transmitted to his or her offspring. If errors in chromosomal replication or transmission continue to occur in the somatic cells, the affected individual's phenotype may change over time.

CHROMOSOMAL ALTERATIONS IN GERM CELLS

Abnormalities of chromosomal transmission: nondisjunction. The chromosomal mechanism that explains the acquisition of an extra chromosome 21 in Down syndrome is called, *nondisjunction.*[1] In this process two chromosomes of a pair are carried to one pole of a dividing nucleus; thus, one daughter cell inherits two chromosomes of a pair and the other daughter cell inherits none. When fertilized with a normal gamete, the resulting offspring has either a trisomy or a monosomy (Fig. 4.3).

Most cases of Down syndrome and other trisomies and monosomies occur as sporadic events; however, the overall occurrence of nondisjunction in gametes is high. Cytogenetic surveys of fetuses aborted during the first trimester of pregnancy have demonstrated that approximately one-third to one-half have trisomies or monosomies.[8-11] The viable conditions include monosomy X, trisomy 21, and

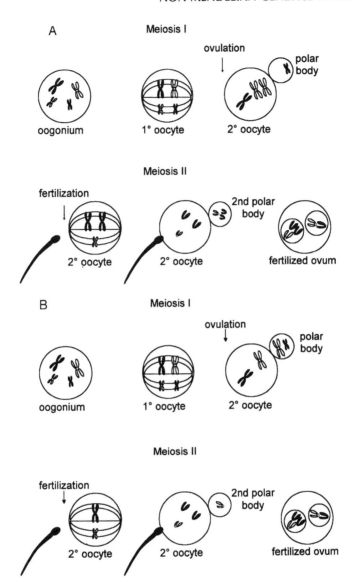

Figure 4.3. Chromosomal nondisjunction in somatic cells, during meiosis I (A) and during meiosis II (B). MI errors lead to copies of the two different chromosomes in the germ cells, whereas MII errors lead to two copies of the same chromosome in the germ cells.

sex chromosome trisomies (Table 4.1).[12–14] Although trisomies 13 and 18 are frequently carried to term, infants with these conditions usually die during the first year of life as a result of the severe congenital malformations. Other trisomies are generally lethal before birth.

The timing of nondisjunction in male or female gametes is variable, occurring

Table 4.1. Viability of Chromosomal Trisomies

Viable in nonmosaic state [141]	Viable with confined placental mosaicism [142]	Viable with somatic mosaicism and/or confined placental mosaicism [141,142]	Mostly inviable: Occasionally viable with somatic mosaicism and/or confined placental mosaicism [141–143]
21	13	8	1
X	18	9	2
Y		12	3
		20	4
		22	5
			6
			7
			11
			14
			15
			16
			17
			19

either during the first or the second stage of meiosis. In approximately 95% of sporadic, nondisjunctional trisomy 21, the extra chromosome 21 is maternal in origin, and in at least 80% of these cases the nondisjunctional error occurs in meiosis I.[15,16] This occurs with increased frequency in the gametes of older mothers. The occurrence of nondisjunction in maternal germ cells reflects information about the physical state of the chromosomes during gamete development. A majority of cases are associated with decreased recombination or failure of any recombination to occur between the two chromosomes.[4,16,17] This may indicate that during the stage of crossing over, the two chromosomes do not pair. The remaining maternal cases and the paternal cases may result from physical alteration of the mitotic spindles that pulls chromosomes apart during the first or second cell divisions. Physical attachment of the chromosomes or unequal force from one side of the spindle may cause both chromosomes to be pulled to the same pole.

Usually nondisjunction is a sporadic process and the child with Down syndrome is the only affected member in the family; however, families have been described in which more than one case of nondisjunction has occurred, resulting in trisomy.[18,19] In several studies of families with recurrent trisomy 21, analysis of chromosomes in the parents' white cells indicated that one of the parents had a normal cell line and a second cell line with trisomy 21 *(somatic mosaicism)*.[16,20] Although some individuals with somatic mosaicism for trisomy 21 have Down syndrome, the level of mosaicism in the parent is generally insufficient to produce this condition. Nevertheless, the chromosomal mosaicism is inferred to be present in the germ cells of that parent *(gonadal mosaicism)*; thus, during meiosis, three chromosomes paired, and two were carried to one pole. The observation of increased risk of trisomy 21 in the offspring of women with Down syndrome supports the idea that an extra chromosome 21 in the germ cells is being transmitted.

A. Balanced

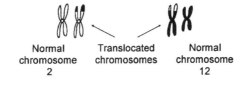

Normal   Translocated   Normal
chromosome   chromosomes   chromosome
2   12

B. Unbalanced

Normal   Translocated Normal   Normal   Translocated Normal
chromosome chromosome chromosomes   chromosomes chromosome chromosome
2   12   2   12

Figure 4.4. Chromosomal translocations may be balanced, resulting in no net gain or loss of genetic information (A), or unbalanced, in which there is a net loss or gain (B).

An increased risk of nondisjunction has been also inferred for the offspring of fertile men with an extra Y chromosome. (This constitution is termed *47,XYY.*) However, this speculation was refuted by direct cytogenetic analysis of sperm from a 47,XYY,[21] although two Y chromosomes tend to be transmitted through meiotic prophase and metaphase I.[22] These cases demonstrate that the extra chromosome may be lost during the process of germ cell maturation or that the presence of an extra chromosome cell may reduce the viability of a maturing germ cell.

Abnormalities of chromosomal segregation: translocations. Physical rearrangement of chromosomes may cause them to be transmitted in a non-Mendelian, but predictable, way. Translocations are rearrangements that occur as the result of breaks in each of two different chromosomes with subsequent joining of the noncontiguous ends (Fig. 4.4). In a number of cases in which the breakpoints of the translocated chromosomes have been identified, the sites of recombination were shown to be both homologous and nonhomologous.[23–25] In one case in which nonhomologous recombination had occurred, short stretches of DNA with similar sequences were found near the site of recombination. If the chromosomal constitution is such that there has been no net loss or gain of information, the translocation is considered to be balanced. If the net information has changed, the translocation is unbalanced.

If a balanced translocation does not disrupt a gene, usually there is no perceptible change in the phenotype. If the translocation interrupts a gene or places it under the control of novel regulatory elements, the translocation can produce an aberrant phenotype, which may be recognizable as a Mendelian phenotype (Fig. 4.5). Translocations have been observed to produce such Mendelian phenotypes as Duchenne muscular dystrophy,[23] neurofibromatosis I,[26] Goltz and Aicardi syndromes,[27] and Menkes disease.[28]

Unbalanced translocations produce variant phenotypes by changing the

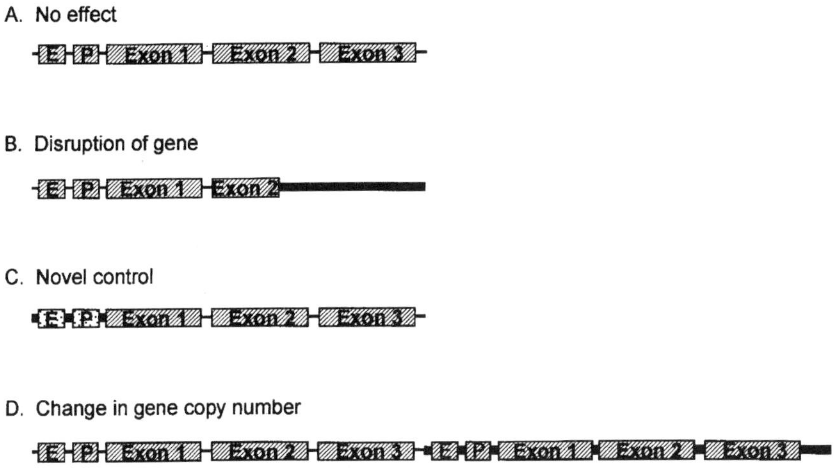

A. No effect

B. Disruption of gene

C. Novel control

D. Change in gene copy number

Figure 4.5. Effects of chromosomal translocations. Chromosomal translocation may produce no effect (A); disrupt a gene, causing premature termination (B); be placed under the control of a novel promoter (C); or change in copy number (D).

gene copy number through deletion or duplication, as well as by interrupting genes and putting the genes under the control of new regulatory elements. Potentially both the duplicated and deleted chromosomal regions contribute to the phenotype, although one may be more overriding than the other. For example, the deletion of one of the short arms of chromosome 17 may produce isolated lissencephaly (smooth brain) despite the fact that there may be a duplicated segment for another chromosome.[29] This suggests that no genes are present in these duplicate regions or that dosage alterations of genes in these regions do not affect the phenotype in ways that have been recognized.

Translocations are not transmitted through the germ line in the usual Mendelian fashion. Ordinarily, chromosomes pair during the diplotene stage of meiosis. If a translocation is present, the two translocated partners align with their two normal homologues in a structure that is termed a *quadrivalent.* Several different forms of transmission can occur from these paired forms into the daughter cells. These are termed alternating, adjacent-1, adjacent-2, and 3:1 (Fig. 4.6). Alternate segregation means that the two translocated chromosomes migrate to one daughter gamete and that the two normal chromosomes migrate to the other daughter gamete (Fig. 4.6A). When these gametes fuse with normal gametes during fertilization, the resulting zygotes have balanced chromosomal constitutions with either a normal set of chromosomes or a translocated set of chromosomes like one of the parents.

Adjacent segregation means that one normal chromosome and one translocated chromosome migrate to different gametes. Adjacent-1 segregation refers to two chromosomes with different centromeres migrating to the same gametes (Fig. 4.6B), whereas adjacent-2 segregation refers to two chromosomes with

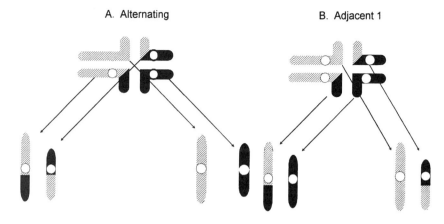

A. Alternating
B. Adjacent 1

Result: balanced gametes
Result: unbalanced gametes

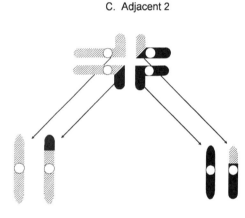

C. Adjacent 2

Result: unbalanced gametes

Figure 4.6. Segregation of chromo-somal translocations. In alternate segregation the two translocated chromosomes migrate to one daughter gamete and the two nor-mal chromosomes migrate to the other daughter gamete (A). Adja-cent segregation means that one normal chromosome and one translocated chromosome migrate to the same gametes. Adjacent-1 segregation refers to two chromo-somes with different centromeres migrating to the same gametes (B), whereas adjacent-2 segregation re-fers to two chromosomes with the same centromere migrating to the same gametes (C).

the same centromeres migrating to the same gametes (Fig. 4.6C). When the gametes that are produced from adjacent segregation fuse with normal gametes during fertilization, the resulting zygotes have unbalanced chromosomal consti-tutions with both duplicated and deleted segments.

A rare form of segregation is termed 3:1. In this case, three chromosomes in the paired quadrivalent set migrate to one gamete and one chromosome mi-grates to the other. When these fuse with normal gametes during fertilization, the resulting zygotes have an unbalanced chromosomal constitution.

From studying the chromosomal constitution of zygotes, it has been discov-ered that the frequency of all of the possible gametes, balanced and unbalanced, is not equal.[30,31] First, this may indicate that the different forms of segregation do not occur with equal frequency. Second, selection may occur at the gamete level, with some types of gametes being inviable. For example, egg precursor cells missing part of the second X chromosome may regress more rapidly.[32]

Third, selection may occur at the zygote level. Some zygotes that have unbalanced chromosomal constitutions may not be implanted or, if implanted, may be spontaneously aborted during the pregnancy.

As judged by chromosome surveys of live-born infants, certain constitutional chromosomal abnormalities are never observed, suggesting that they are not compatible with gestation.[12–14] Some of these nonviable chromosomal abnormalities are observed in fetuses spontaneously aborted during the first trimester of pregnancy, confirming the idea of nonviability.[33] Others are not observed even in first-trimester abortuses, suggesting even earlier lethality (Table 4.1).

The frequency of offspring with the various phenotypes that are produced by translocation carriers does not follow Mendelian transmission. Rather, the frequency of their occurrence must be determined empirically. Based on these empiric observations, efforts have been made to develop algorithms to predict the likelihood of these events.[30,34]

Abnormalities of recombination. Another way in which chromosomal transmission can be altered is by unequal recombination. This process involves pairing between chromosomes in which each chromosome has at least two copies of homologous genes in a tandem array. Through the process of unequal recombination, the gene copy number is altered or hybrid genes are formed with novel properties.

The frequency with which new unequal recombinational events occurs between the X and Y chromosomes is approximately 1:30,000.[25,35] The frequencies of the unequal recombinational events that are associated with copy number polymorphisms in the α-globin and X-linked cone opsin gene loci are unknown; however, based on analysis of linked polymorphisms, the unequal recombinational events of the cone opsin loci have occurred a number of times.[36]

Structural variation of chromosomes can increase the frequency of unequal recombination. One such example is that of chromosome inversions in which abnormal recombinational events occur (Fig. 4.7). The inversions may be of two types, paracentric, that is, involving both sides of the centromere,[37,38] and pericentric,[39] that is, involving only one side. Paracentric chromosomes form inversion loops to pair with their normal homologues. If crossing over occurs outside the inversion loop, no abnormal products are formed. If the breakage and recombination occur within the loop, the products have both duplicated and deleted segments, a phenomenon that has been called *recombination aneusomy*.[40] Depending on the size of the duplicated and deleted regions in the offspring, the phenotype may be abnormal. The sites of recombination may vary from one gamete to another, so each offspring may seem a sporadic case with a novel phenotype.

To pair with their normal homologues during meiosis, chromosomes with pericentric inversions also form inversion loops.[39] If crossing over occurs outside the inversion loop, no abnormal products are formed. If recombination occurs within the inversion loop, two types of products are formed, acentric fragments and dicentric chromosomes. Acentric fragments do not have a centromere and are lost during mitosis.

Dicentric chromosomes may be unstable in germ or somatic cells if both centromeres are active.[41] Under some circumstances, when both centromeres are active, the unequal force of the mitotic spindle on each of the centromeres can pull the chromosomes apart, resulting in transmission of different chromosomal fragments to the daughter cells. The chromosomal fragments may be acentric. The fragments may have a single active centromere, and unless incorporated into another chromosome, may be transmitted faithfully. Alternatively, the chromosomal fragments may have two active centromeres and be subject to further fragmentation. As a

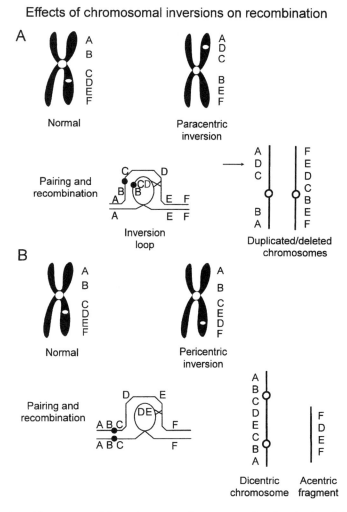

Figure 4.7. Chromosomal inversions may be paracentric, that is, involving both sides of the centromere (A) or pericentric, that is, involving only one side (B). Pairing and recombination of paracentric inversions leads to the formation of duplicated and deleted chromosomes. Pairing and recombination of pericentric inversions leads to the formation of dicentric chromosomes of acentric fragments.

result, the progeny cells of those containing dicentric chromosomes may have different genetic constitutions and different phenotypes.

CHROMOSOMAL ALTERATIONS IN SOMATIC CELLS

Altered chromosomal constitution. Zygotes may start off with a normal complement of chromosomes, but as a result of errors in transmission or replication in somatic cells, the mature organism may have cells with altered chromosomal constitutions. These cells are usually not observed and do not produce phenotypic effects unless the level of somatic mosaicism is high enough to affect a significant proportion of the cells. Generally, there are two ways in which this can happen. First, the chromosomal mosaicism may occur in the embryo and affect the development of the organism. Second, the chromosomal mosaicism may occur later in development but confer a growth advantage to the cells with the abnormal chromosomal constitution. Such growth advantage is observed in malignancies and in conditions of benign overgrowth.

One of the first clues that chromosomal alterations occurred in somatic cells was the observation of a chromosomal variant in chronic myelogenous leukemia (CML) that was called the Philadelphia-1 (Ph^1) chromosome.[42] The high rate of occurrence of this chromosomal variant in CML became a diagnostic criterion for the disorder. When chromosomal banding studies became available, it was shown that this variant was the result of a balanced translocation between chromosomes 9 and 22.[43] When molecular cloning techniques became available, it was shown that the sites of recombination of this variant occurred within a fairly short interval on these two chromosomes that always involved two genes, the c-abl oncogene on chromosome 22 and the bcr (for breakpoint cluster region on chromosome 9).[43–45] The effect of this translocation was to put the c-abl gene under the control of the bcr region, thereby conferring novel properties.

Consistent patterns of translocations were found in other tumors as well. Translocations involving chromosome 8 were found in virtually all Burkitt lymphomas, a tumor of-B cell origin. The most common of these translocations involved chromosome 14,[46,47] although translocations involving chromosomes 2 and 22 were also identified.[48] The site of translocation on chromosome 8 always involved the c-myc oncogene, whereas the sites on the other chromosomes involved the genes for the immunoglobulin heavy-chain (chromosome 14) and light-chain genes (κ chain—chromosome 2, and λ chain—chromosome 22).[49–52]

These patterns suggested that the recombinational machinery of the B cells was involved in the formation of the translocations. Ordinarily the immunoglobulin genes undergo a process of somatic recombination in which different gene segments contribute to the formation of the mature gene and its transcript. This process involves a recombinase and a series of recognition sites either seven or nine bases in length that are present on the 5' side of the regions of the immunoglobulin genes to be joined.[53–55] These sites are present in other regions of the genome including on the 5' side of the myc oncogene. When the repeats adjacent to the c-myc oncogene pair with those of the immunoglobulin genes, recombination takes place. These translocations have two effects. First,

the c-myc oncogene is placed under the control of the immunoglobulin en-
hancer, altering the expression of this gene. Second, a repressor in the c-myc
oncogene is lost as a result of the translocation.

Abnormalities of chromosomal organization in somatic cells involve not only
translocations but also deletions. Among the first examples to be identified were
deletions of chromosome 13 in individuals with sporadic cases of retinoblastoma[56,57] and of chromosome 11 in sporadic cases of Wilms tumor.[58] By contrast, in some familial cases of both of these conditions, germline deletions
were found in all of the cells of the affected individual.[59,60] Moreover, individuals who had germline deletions were far more likely to have multiple tumors
in one or both organs.[61] These findings suggested that dose-dependent tumor
suppressor genes may be located within these chromosomal regions.

Abnormalities of chromosomal transmission. Abnormalities in chromosomal transmission occur because chromosomes are lost or gained in somatic
cells or because the chromosomes have unstable structures that result in their
being fragmented or lost. Chromosomal nondisjunction occurs in the somatic
cells of normal zygotes, resulting in monosomy or trisomy. For example, Down
syndrome may be the effect of nondisjunction in somatic cells as well as in
germ cells.[62,63] If the postzygotic nondisjunction occurs early and the level of
chromosomal mosaicism is high, the phenotypes may be indistinguishable from
those that occur from nondisjunction in germ cells.

Chromosomal gain or loss may also result in early embryos with abnormal
chromosomal constitutions and may have the effect of "correcting" these chromosomal abnormalities.[62,64] Thus, embryos that were originally monosomic or
trisomic may appear to have normal chromosomal constitutions in most of their
cells. Distinguishing between postzygotic errors and postzygotic correction of
errors in gamete transmission may be difficult. In some cases where both chromosomes in the normal karyotype originate from one parent, the individual's
phenotype may be abnormal (see Uniparental Disomy).[65] Identifying postzygotic abnormalities of chromosomal transmission requires identifying
populations of cells with abnormal chromosomal constitutions in an individual.

As judged by the number of aneuploid cells (that is, cells with other than 46
chromosomes with 22 pairs of normal autosomes and two normal sex chromosomes), the frequency of chromosomal nondisjunction increases with age. Certain aneuploid states are commonly seen with increasing age, for example, loss
of a Y chromosome in male somatic cells and loss of the second X chromosome
in female somatic cells.[66,67] These aneuploid states have no demonstrable phenotypic consequences.

Chromosomal nondisjunction may be more readily observed in certain per-
missive genetic backgrounds, for example, in tumor cells. Presumably the genetic changes in these cells have caused them to become immortalized and less
sensitive to loss or gain of a chromosome. Cytogenetic studies of ovarian cancer have demonstrated marked variability in the chromosomal constitution of
the tumors, including modal numbers that are hypodiploid (less than 40 chro-

mosomes) or hyperdiploid (60 to 100 chromosomes), the presence of multiple chromosomal markers, and the presence of cells with spontaneous chromosome breaks.[68–70]

Certain chromosomal structures are unstable and are not faithfully transmitted to daughter cells. As discussed previously, the most salient example is that of dicentric chromosomes, in which two centromeres are present on one chromosome. These two centromeres may have originated from different chromosomes via a translocation. Alternatively, the two centromeres may have originated from the same chromosome through the process of unequal recombination.

UNIPARENTAL DISOMY

One unusual form of chromosomal transmission is called *uniparental disomy*.[65,71,72] Humans with uniparental disomy have two copies of a chromosome or of a chromosomal region from one parent and no copies from the other. Two types of uniparental disomy have been identified—isodisomy, in which there is inheritance of two copies of the identical chromosome from one parent,[65] and heterodisomy, in which there is inheritance of the parent's two different chromosomes.[73] Depending on the region involved, this may produce new phenotypic effects. Several different mechanisms, both prezygotic and postzygotic, have been postulated to cause uniparental isodisomy in humans (Fig. 4.8).[71] These may involve errors in chromosomal transmission or errors in recombination.

Errors of chromosomal transmission. Some gametes lack a chromosome. If uncorrected, the resulting monosomy in the zygote would be lethal. Correction occurs when the other gamete of the zygote has two copies of the deficient chromosome or when that gamete has one copy, but it is duplicated in the zygote. These processes are collectively known as *gamete complementation* (Fig. 4.8A). A variant of the process is postzygotic loss of a chromosome followed by duplication of the remaining chromosome in the pair. Another way for uniparental disomy to occur is for one gamete to contribute two chromosomes and the other gamete to contribute one chromosome of that pair. Subsequent, nondisjunctional loss of a chromosome in the zygote results in some cells having uniparental disomy (Fig. 4.8A).

Errors of somatic recombination. Other mechanisms that can produce uniparental disomy are somatic recombination and gene conversion (Fig. 4.8B).[74] Depending on the segregation of the chromatids at meiosis, the region distal to a given site of recombination will be identical in the daughter cells. As a result of gene conversion, all of the sequences within a given region of both chromosomes in a daughter cells will be identical. As with other events involving chromosomal mosaicism, the proportion of cells that have uniparental disomy depends on the time in development when the genetic event occurred and the fitness of the daughter cells.

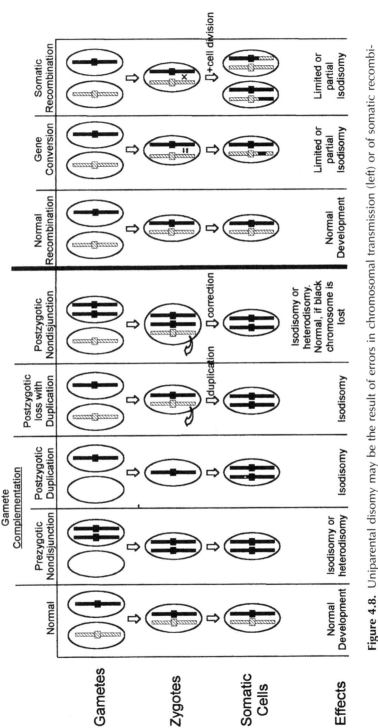

Figure 4.8. Uniparental disomy may be the result of errors in chromosomal transmission (left) or of somatic recombination (right). These may produce isodisomy, in which there is inheritance of two copies of the identical chromosome from one parent, or heterodisomy, in which there is inheritance of the parent's two different chromosomes.[71]

Judith Hall has suggested that uniparental disomy may be a common occurrence in humans.[75] She postulated that up to 1% of human conceptions may start with chromosomal trisomies that spontaneously "correct" postzygotically to uniparental disomy, thereby preventing antenatal lethality. This hypothesis was supported by the relatively high frequency of chromosomal mosaicism in human chorionic villi (2.5%);[76] however, there has not been independent ascertainment of the frequency of uniparental disomy in human populations.

The mechanisms of uniparental disomy may influence the observed phenotype (Table 4.2). First, the proportion of cells that have uniparental disomy may contribute to the phenotype; thus, some cells may be diploid whereas others are aneuploid. Second, the phenotype may be affected by the presence of two different uniparental alleles as opposed to the presence of two copies of the same allele. Third, the allele inherited from one parent may be inactive or differentially expressed compared to the allele inherited from the other parent; thus, the affected individual may have cells with two active or two inactive alleles when one allele would be expressed ordinarily. This phenomenon appears to be the case for Beckwith-Wiedemann syndrome, a condition associated with overgrowth of the tongue and the abdominal viscera. The somatic overgrowth can be explained by the presence of two active insulin-like growth factor 2 genes, whereas normally, individuals have one active and one inactive gene (a phenomenon that is called *genomic imprinting*—see chapter 7).[77,78]

Uniparental disomy has been found in individuals with a readily discerned autosomal recessive condition with atypical features. For example, two individuals were described with cystic fibrosis and intrauterine growth retardation. Both had maternal isodisomy of chromosome 7.[71,72] In each case, nonpaternity was excluded by analysis of multiple DNA markers. These findings in multiple individuals suggest that the intrauterine growth retardation could be explained on the basis of the uniparental disomy. Another individual with homozygous deficiency of complement C4 and systemic lupus erythematosus had paternal isodisomy for chromosome 6.[79] Only the transmitting parent was likely to be heterozygous for the autosomal recessive condition.

Uniparental disomy for other chromosomes has been associated with abnormal phenotypes that were not associated with various Mendelian conditions.

Table 4.2 Uniparental disomy associated with a specific phenotype

Chromosome	Phenotype
7mat	Growth retardation [71,72]
11pat	Beckwith-Wiedeman syndrome [144]
14mat	Short stature, precocious puberty, arrested hydrocephalus, small hands and feet, delayed motor and /or mental development [80,81]
15mat	Prader-Willi syndrome [73]
15pat	Angelman syndrome [145–147]

Maternal heterodisomy for chromosome 14 was observed in a boy with hydrocephalus, bifid uvula, premature puberty, short stature, and small testes.[80] On the other hand, paternal uniparental heterodisomy for chromosome 14 was found in a girl with a small thoracic cage, marked angulation of the ribs, bilateral subdural hygromas, coarse facial features with frontal bossing, and prominent maxilla and mandible.[81] A child with developmental delay, dolichocephaly, pointed chin, broad nasal bridge, large ears, and sensorineural hearing loss was homozygous for a maternally transmitted chromosome 4 with a pericentric inversion, suggesting maternal isodisomy.[82] Despite the fact that cases with these phenotypic features had not been previously described, they may represent homozygosity for a recessive allele that was inherited from a carrier parent. Alternatively, they may represent cryptic chromosomal trisomies or over- or under-expression of an imprinted gene.

Some cases of uniparental disomy are associated with normal phenotypes. Two individuals with maternal uniparental disomy for chromosome 22 were phenotypically normal.[83,84] These case suggests that it is unlikely that parental origin influences the expression of genes on chromosome 22.

LOSS OF HETEROZYGOSITY

Chromosomal alterations that result in the development of human tumors may be inherited in the germ line or may represent somatic changes in single genes or in chromosomal regions that contain those genes. Based on the distribution of inherited versus sporadic tumors, Alfred Knudson postulated that two genetic hits were required for retinoblastoma and Wilms tumor to develop.[85–87] The effect of these hits was to knock out both copies of a tumor suppressor gene that prevented the development of tumors. In inherited cases, one of the hits was transmitted through the germ line and the other was acquired in the somatic cell. In sporadic cases, both hits occurred in the somatic cell.

By comparing the pattern of polymorphic DNA markers from blood and from tumor tissue, Webster Cavenee and co-workers demonstrated how these two hits occur. Cavenee created the phrase *loss of heterozygosity* to describe his observation of the loss of at least one of the wild-type markers in a specific chromosomal location in tumors (Fig. 4.9).[88] As noted, deletion of chromosome 13 in the region of the retinoblastoma gene can be one hit. The second hit may involve an event that knocked out the function of the remaining wild-type gene, including deletion or insertion. Alteratively, the second hit may involve loss of a chromosome 13 with or without duplication of the deletion-bearing chromosome 13. Other mechanisms involve somatic recombination between the chromatids of the wild type and deletion-bearing chromosomes or mutation limited to the wild type allele.

The identification of loss of heterozygosity suggested that the development of retinoblastoma and Wilms and other tumors constituted recessive phenotypes because two hits were required for the tumor to develop.[88,89] This explained

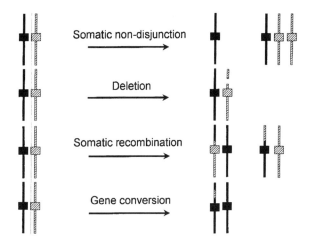

Figure 4.9. Genetic mechanisms that result in loss of heterozygosity for chromosomal markers.

why some individuals who inherited an allele for retinoblastoma did not develop the disease. This nonpenetrance resulted from the absence of a second hit. It also suggested the mechanism of action for Rb and other genes. In the wild type, these acted as tumor suppressor genes. With loss or complete inactivation, tumors could develop. With the identification of the Rb protein, this mechanism of action was proven to be correct.[90]

Osteogenic sarcomas were observed in individuals who survived retinoblastoma.[91,92] Initially these tumors were thought to be the result of treatment with radiation and/or chemotherapy. Detailed analysis demonstrated that the same genetic mechanism operates in the bone and the retina. Loss of heterozygosity was demonstrated in osteogenic sarcomas, although the loss occurs preferentially for the paternal alleles.[93] The molecular basis of this difference is not yet understood. Loss of heterozygosity for the Rb gene has been found to play a role in other tumors, including small-cell carcinoma of the lung.[94] This demonstrates that one cancer-causing gene can have an effect on the development of many other tumors. Loss of heterozygosity has been implicated in the development and progression of a host of other tumors, including common solid tumors such as those of colon, lung, and breast.[95,96]

CONSEQUENCES OF ABNORMAL CHROMOSOMAL TRANSMISSION

Constitutional. Constitutional chromosomal changes (i.e., affecting all of the cells in the body) may have no phenotypic effects at all. Balanced translocation carriers and individuals with 47,XXY chromosomal constitutional may not be identified until they have chromosome analysis performed as part of an infertility workup or for some other reason.

Alternatively, constitutional chromosomal changes may be associated with one or more Mendelian phenotypes because disruption, loss, or novel control of a gene resulted in a Mendelian phenotype. When more than one gene is disrupted, two or more Mendelian phenotypes may be produced. This condition is known as a *contiguous gene syndrome.*[97] One of the first individuals with a contiguous gene syndrome to be recognized had a deletion of the short arm of his X chromosome.[98] This produced Duchenne muscular dystrophy, retinitis pigmentosa, chronic granulomatous disease, and the McLeod blood group. Other examples of contiguous gene syndromes are listed in Table 4.3.

Constitutional chromosomal disorders also produce recognizable syndromes. These are associated with unbalanced karyotypes and quantitative alterations in gene expression. Limited or critical regions of chromosomes may be sufficient to produce these conditions. For example, trisomy for the whole of chromosome 21 is not necessary to produce Down syndrome. Individuals with duplications of the distal long arm of chromosome 21, resulting in three copies of band q22, have a condition that is indistinguishable from that of individuals with true trisomy 21.[99] Other chromosomal constitutions that produce the Down syndrome phenotype include trisomy 21q based on a translocation involving the long arms of chromosome 21 and another acrocentric chromosome *(Robertsonian translocation)* or chromosomal mosaicism (46,XY/47,XY+21).[100–102]

Phenotypic characteristics of constitutional chromosomal abnormalities. There are certain phenotypic characteristics of the recognizable syndromes that are produced by constitutional chromosomal abnormalities. First, greater than 90% of constitutional chromosomal abnormalities do not survive to term, even for the trisomy 21 and monosomy X that are observed in newborns.[103,104] If viable, multiple systems tend to be involved, including the central nervous system. Mental retardation is a common abnormality. The longevity of individuals with these conditions tends to be reduced. The fertility of affected individuals also tends to be reduced. For certain chromosomal disorders, such as trisomy 21, 46,XY gonadal dysgenesis, and deletions of the long arm of chromosome 13 and the short arm of chromosome 11, the risk of malignancy is increased.[58,61,105,106]

Constitutional chromosomal abnormalities and variable expressivity. Constitutional chromosomal abnormalities that appear to be similar on karyotype analysis may differ when analyzed for their phenotypic effects. First, precise molecular analysis may show that some individuals have single-gene conditions, whereas others have different contiguous gene syndromes. For example, depending on the size of the deletion of the short arm of the X chromosome, individuals may have one or more of the following conditions: steroid sulfatase deficiency, Kallman syndrome, chondrodysplasia punctata, optic albinism, adrenal hypoplasia, glycerol kinase deficiency, and Duchenne muscular dystrophy.[27,107] Second, there can be somatic progression of a constitutional chromo-

Table 4.3. Contiguous gene syndromes

Chromosomal region	Phenotype
3q12-q23	Blepharophimosis, ptosis, epicanthus inversus[148]
5p-	Cri-du-chat[149]
8p11.23-p21.1	Spherocytosis, mental retardation, multiple congenital anomalies[150]
8q12-q21.2	Duane syndrome, branchio-otorenal syndrome, hydrocephalus[151]
8q-	Langer-Gideon syndrome (trichorhino-phalangeal dysplasia ± multiple exostoses)[152]
11p13	Wilms tumor—aniridia[58,153]
15q11-q13	Prader-Willi, hypopigmentation[154,155]
15q11-q13	Angelman, hypopigmentation[156]
16p13	Infantile polycystic kidney—tuberous sclerosis[157]
16p13.3	Alpha-thalassemia—mental retardation[158]
17p13.3	Miller-Dieker (lissencephaly +)[159]
18q-	Growth retardation, microcephaly, facial dysmorphism, hypoplastic genitalia, limb anomalies, hypotonia, deafness[160]
22q11	DiGeorge or velocardiofacial or CHARGE (Coloboma, Heart anomaly, Choanal Atresia, Genital, and Ear anomalies) associations[161–163]
Xp22.31	Goltz and Aicadi syndromes, steroid sulfatase deficiency, Kallman syndrome, chondrodysplasia punctata, ocular albinism
Xp21	Glycerol kinase deficiency, Duchenne muscular dystrophy, adrenal hypoplasia congenita, chronic granulomatous disease, retinitis pigmentosa, McLeod blood group[98,164]
Xp11.3	Norrie disease and monoamine oxidase deficiency[165]
Xq21	Adrenal leukodystrophy, color vision deficiencies[166]

somal abnormality, as occurs, for instance, with isodicentric chromosomes. Third, there can be a parental origin effect. The consequences of uniparental disomy for the long arm of chromosome 15 (Angelman or Prader-Willi syndrome) differ depending on whether this is maternally or paternally inherited (see chapter 7).

Phenotypic characteristics of somatic mosaicism. Besides its effect in producing cancers and somatic overgrowth, somatic mosaicism can affect the development of the organism in several ways. Frequently, somatic mosaicism results in a milder phenotype than a constitutional abnormality. The physical abnormalities may be limited to a single (or at most a few) organ systems. For example, trisomy 21 that is confined to the bone marrow in the newborn is not associated with any of the physical stigmata of Down syndrome. Rather, the infant has an elevated number of circulating white blood cells, known as a leukemoid reaction. This may progress to leukemia or may be self-limited and regress.[108,109]

Somatic mosaicism can produce characteristic pigmentary alterations. Typically, these are regions of hypo- or hyperpigmentation that follow a distribution along the lines of Blaschko, lines that simulate the migrational patterns of pigmentary cells from the somites of the embryo.[110] These are classified as hypomelanosis of Ito if the hypopigmented areas follow Blaschko's lines, or as linear and whorled hypermelanosis if hyperpigmented areas follow this distribution.[111] Chromosomal studies of skin fibroblasts have shown that either the hypopigmented or the hyperpigmented skin may have one or more cell types with abnormal chromosomal constitutions.[112–115] Many different chromosomes have been found in the fibroblasts of the abnormally pigmented skin, suggesting that many genes play a role in the normal pigmentation process.

Some of the recognizable syndromes with abnormal pigmentation as a characteristic feature have somatic overgrowth, tumors, mental retardation, and reduced viability as other characteristic features. Rudolf Happle suggested that these conditions were the result of somatic mosaicism and may not be viable in the nonmosaic state.[116] This assumption of improved viability has been inferred for disorders that have been observed only in the mosaic state. These include trisomy 8 and Pallister-Killian syndrome, a condition associated with mosaic tetrasomy for the short arm of chromosome 12.[117,118]

Somatic mosaicism confined to the placenta. A special case is that of chromosomal mosaicism confined to the placenta (Table 4.4). In these cases, chromosomal alterations are found in the placenta that are not found in other somatic tissues.[119] In cases of trisomies 13 and 18, confined placental mosaicism for a *normal* cell line has been correlated with viability at birth for infants who otherwise were found to have true autosomal trisomies.[120] Conversely, cell lines with abnormal chromosomal constitutions confined to the placenta have been found in cases of in utero growth retardation in infants who otherwise had normal somatic chromosomal constitutions.[121] The findings suggest that chromosomal mosaicism affects the function of the placenta and may in turn contribute to the development of the fetus. In contrast, confined placental mosaicism for a normal cell line is not an apparent requirement for viability in fetuses with trisomy 21.[120]

Table 4.4. Placental Chromosomal Mosaicism in Viable Conceptions with Trisomies 13, 18, and 21[120]

Chromosomal aneuploidy	Placental tissue		Amnion culture	Fetal tissue	
	Cytotrophoblast direct prep	Villus stroma culture		Chorion culture	Cord blood or tissue
Trisomy 13	+	−	−	−	−
Trisomy 18	+	−	−	−	−
Trisomy 21	−	−	−	−	−

Somatic mosaicism in monozygotic twins. Chromosomal mosaicism can affect monozygotic twins, causing them to have discordant phenotypes. For example, monozygotic twins have been identified who were discordant for their sexual development.[122–124] Detailed analysis in one pair was illustrative of the effects of mosaicism.[123] The male twin had a 46,XY karyotype and normal development. The female twin had a 45,X karyotype and the phenotype of Turner syndrome. Analysis of zygosity using polymorphic DNA markers showed that the fetuses were the product of a single zygote with subsequent twinning. Neither of the twins had chromosomal mosaicism in their tissues; however, analysis of blood showed that both had two populations of cells, with 45,X and 46,XY karyotypes. The twinning process and the chromosomal nondisjunction occurred close to one another in time, so each twin had a homogenous population of cells in his or her tissues. The mixed population of cells in the blood was explained as the result of twin–twin transfusion during gestation.

Somatic mosaicism for single gene mutations. Somatic mosaicism can occur for mutations in single genes. If enough cells are affected, the somatic mosaicism can produce abnormal Mendelian phenotypes. Usually, these are milder or have a focal distribution. For example, a male with ornithine transcarbamylase (OTC) deficiency, whose disease did not become apparent until later in childhood, was found to have somatic mosaicism for a mutation in his OTC gene.[125] The disease became apparent only after a febrile illness produced a severe endogenous catabolic protein load. Somatic mosaicism for a mutation in the stimulatory subunit of the GTP-binding protein causes the McCune-Albright syndrome, a condition that is characterized by café-au-lait spots on the skin, a fibrous dysplasia affecting multiple bones, and a polyendocrinopathy in which the end-organs are overresponsive to the effects of polypeptide hormones.[126] Normally, the GTP-binding protein acts as a second messenger for several polypeptide hormones, including TSH, LH, FSH, ACTH, and PTH (thyroid stimulating hormone, luteinizing hormone, follicle stimulating hormone, adrenocortical trophic hormone and parathyroid hormone). As the result of overstimulation of the gonads by gonadotrophins, precocious puberty is common in this condition. If such a mutation were present in the nonmosaic state, it would probably be lethal.[127]

Although somatic mutation may occur with increased frequency in conditions with abnormal somatic replication, the basal rate human cells, as judged by mutations in the glycophorin and HPRT gene, is 10.$^{-5}$ to 10^{-6}.[128,129] Assuming that there are 10^{13}–10^{14} cells in the human body, it is likely that the entire repertoire of known mutations occurs during embryonic, fetal, or extrauterine life. The cells in which these mutations occur may be inviable or may occur too late in the life cycle of the individual to reach a threshold to produce phenotypic effects. Nonetheless, all cancers are associated with somatic mutation; thus, somatic mosaicism is observed in the 25–30% of the population that develops cancer.

Gonadal mosaicism. Mosaicism may occur in germ cells as well as somatic cells. Depending on the time when a chromosomal alteration or single mutation occurs, multiple germ cells may be affected. During fetal life there are 4 million ova in the combined ovaries. Assuming that the mutation rate is 10^{-4}–10^{-7} per locus per gamete,[130,131] and that these occur with equal likelihood in the postulated 50,000–100,000 loci, there may be several ova with mutations for each of the common disorders. Some alterations are unique, whereas others may be clonal if they occurred before the germ cells entered the meiotic pathway. In female germ cells there are 30 mitoses before the first meiotic event.[132] The number of mitotic divisions prior to meiosis is much greater in males. As a result, gonadal mosaicism for multiple disorders may be a feature of each gonad.[7]

Gonadal mosaicism is identified most readily when individuals who have normal somatic genetic constitutions have more than one child with a genetic disorder.[133–135] Usually, the gonadal mosaicism is inferred, although the parent in whom it is present can be identified by linkage analysis using markers in the vicinity of the disease locus.[136] Gonadal mosaicism in the father's germ cells has been proven in a case of osteogenesis imperfecta in which the mutation in the $\alpha 1$ collagen gene was also found in the father's sperm.[137] Gonadal mosaicism is common in Duchenne muscular dystrophy. In about one-third of cases, the mother cannot be demonstrated to be a carrier by genetic testing of her somatic cells. Nonetheless, over 40% of these mothers of sporadic cases may have gonadal mosaicism.[138] In the aggregate the risk that a "noncarrier" mother may have a second affected male child is 14%.[139]

If mutation or chromosomal alteration occurs during early embryonic life, the affected individual may have both somatic and gonadal mosaicism. As with other cases of somatic mosaicism, these individuals may not be identified until they have an affected child. When these individuals are subsequently examined, they may be found to have mild manifestations of the disease. For example, a man who had two children with osteogenesis imperfecta was found to have both gonadal and somatic mosaicism. When questioned, he was found to have had more bone fractures than would have been predicted by chance alone.[140]

CONSEQUENCES OF CHROMOSOMAL TRANSMISSION

The physical basis of Mendelian transmission is the faithful transmission of chromosomes in germ and somatic cells. Aberrant chromosomal transmission can occur in germ or somatic cells. In germ cells, translocations between chromosomes increase the likelihood of aberrant chromosomal transmission. Unfaithful transmission of chromosomes can also result from chromosomal nondisjunction and from abnormalitites of recombination. Certain chromosomal structures such as dicentric chromosomes are unstable. Aberrant chromosomal transmission can produce disease in several ways. Genes can be disrupted from translocation or deletions. Deleterious or imprinted alleles may be unmasked as the result of deletion or uniparental disomy. Some genes, if overexpressed, may produce new phenotypes.

The chromosomal constitution is likely to vary among the cells in any person's body. The presence of somatic mosaicism may result in variable expressivity and even nonpenetrance for a genetic condition within a family. The presence of gonadal mosaicism may result in multiple siblings with a dominant or X-linked condition born to seemingly unaffected or noncarrier parents.

Not every chromosome works in the same way. Sex chromosomes have unique properties that affect their transmission and the expression of their genes. Indeed, sex chromosome transmisison was not predicted by Mendel's laws.

REFERENCES

1. Bridges CB. Non-disjunction as proof of the chromosome theory of heredity. Genetics 1:1–52, 107–163, 1916.
2. Lejeune J, Gautier M, Turpin MR. Etude des chromosome somatiques de neuf enfants mongoliens. CR Acad Sci 248:1721–1722, 1959.
3. Ford CE, Miller OJ, Polani PE. A sex-chromosome anomaly in a case of gonadal dysgenesis (Turner syndrome). Lancet 1:711–713, 1959.
4. Jacobs PA, Strong JA. A case of human intersexuality having a possible XXY sex-determining mechanism. Nature 183:302–303, 1959.
5. Morgan TH, Sturtevant AH, Muller HJ, Bridges CB. The Mechanism of Mendelian Inheritance. New York: Henry Holt, 1915.
6. Panthier JJ, Condamine H. Mitotic recombination in mammals. Bioessays 13:351–356, 1991.
7. Hall JG. Review and hypotheses: somatic mosaicism: observations related to clinical genetics. Am J Hum Genet 43:355–363, 1988.
8. Boue A, Boue J. Evaluation of chromosome errors at the moment of conception. (French). Biomedicine 18:372–374, 1973.
9. Burgoyne PS, Holland K, Stephens R. Incidence of numerical chromosome anomalies in human pregnancy estimation from induced and spontaneous abortion data. Hum Reprod 6:555–565, 1991.
10. Ma S, Kalousek DK, Yuen BH, Gomel V, Katagiri S, Moon YS. Chromosome investigation in *in vitro* fertilization failure. J Assist Reprod Genet 11:445–451, 1994.
11. Macas E, Floersheim Y, Hotz E, Imthurn B, Keller PJ, Walt H. Abnormal chromosomal arrangements in human oocytes. Hum Reprod 5:703–707, 1990.
12. Hamerton JL, Canning N, Ray M, Smith S. A cytogenetic survey of 14,069 newborn infants. I. Incidence of chromosome abnormalities. Clin Genet 8:223–243, 1975.
13. Jacobs PA, Melville M, Ratcliffe S, Keay AJ, Syme J. A cytogenetic survey of 11,680 newborn infants. Ann Hum Genet 37:359–376, 1974.
14. Sergovich F, Valentine GH, Chen AT, Kinch RA, Smout MS. Chromosome aberrations in 2159 consecutive newborn babies. N Engl J Med 280:851–855, 1969.
15. Antonarakis SE, Petersen MB, McInnis MG, Adelsberger PA, Schinzel AA, Binkert F, et al. The meiotic stage of nondisjunction in trisomy 21: determination by using DNA polymorphisms. Am J Hum Genet 50:544–550, 1992.
16. Sherman SL, Petersen MB, Freeman SB, Hersey J, Pettay D, Taft L, et al. Nondisjunction of chromosome 21 in maternal meiosis I: evidence for a maternal age-dependent mechanism involving reduced recombination. Hum Mol Genet 3:1529–1535, 1994.
17. Sherman SL, Takaesu N, Freeman SB, Grantham M, Phillips C, Blackston RD, et al. Trisomy 21: Association between reduced recombination and nondisjunction. Am J Hum Genet 49:608–620, 1991.

18. Sachs ES, Jahoda MG, Los FJ, Pijpers L, Wladimiroff JW. Trisomy 21 mosaicism in gonads with unexpectedly high recurrence risks. Am J Med Genet 7:186–188, 1990.

19. Harris DJ, Begleiter ML, Chamberlin J, Hankins L, Magenis RE. Parental trisomy 21 mosaicism. Am J Hum Genet 34:125–133, 1982.

20. Pangalos CG, Talbot CC, Lewis JG, Adelsberger PA, Petersen MB, Serre JL, et al. DNA polymorphism analysis in families with recurrence of free trisomy 21. Am J Hum Genet 51:1015–1027, 1992.

21. Benet J, Martin RH. Sperm chromosome complements in a 47,XYY man. Hum Genet 78:313–315, 1988.

22. Speed RM, Faed MJ, Batstone PJ, Baxby K, Barnetson W. Persistence of two Y chromosomes through meiotic prophase and metaphase I in an XYY man. Hum Genet 87:416–420, 1991.

23. Worton RG. Duchenne muscular dystrophy: gene and gene product; mechanism of mutation in the gene. (Review). J Inherit Metab Dis 15:539–550, 1992.

24. vanBakel I, Holt S, Craig I, Boyd Y. Sequence analysis of the breakpoint regions of an X;5 translocation in a female with Duchenne muscular dystrophy. Am J Hum Genet 57:329–336, 1995.

25. Petit C, de la Chapelle A, Levilliers J, Castillo S, Noel B, Weissenbach J. An abnormal terminal X-Y interchange accounts for most but not all cases of human XX males. Cell 49:595–602, 1987.

26. Ledbetter DH, Rich DC, O'Connell P, Leppert M, Carey JC. Precise localization of NF1 to 17q11.2 by balanced translocation. Am J Hum Genet 44:20–24, 1989.

27. Ballabio A, Andria G. Deletions and translocations involving the distal short arm of theX human X chromosome: review and hypotheses. Hum Mol Genet 1:221–227, 1992.

28. Mercer JF, Livingston J, Hall B, Paynter JA, Begy C, Chandrasekharappa S, et al. Isolation of a partial candidate gene for Menkes disease by positional cloning. Nat Genet 3:20–25, 1993.

29. Dobyns WB, Truwit CL. Lissencephaly and other malformations of cortical development: 1995 update. (Review). Neuropediatrics 26:132–147, 1995.

30. Jalbert P, Sele B, Jalbert H. Reciprocol translocations: a way to predict the mode of imbalanced segregation by pachytene-diagram drawing. Hum Genet 55:209–222, 1980.

31. Pellestor F, Sele B, Jalbert H, Jalbert P. Direct segregation analysis of reciprocal translocations: a study of 283 sperm karyotypes from four carriers. Am J Hum Genet 44:464–473, 1989.

32. Simpson JL. Abnormal sexual differentiation in humans. Annu Rev Genet 16:193–224, 1982.

33. Boue J, Bou A, Lazar P. Retrospective and prospective epidemiological studies of 1500 karyotyped spontaneous human abortions. Teratology 12:11–26, 1975.

34. Cans C, Cohen O, Mermet MA, Demongeot J, Jalbert P. Human reciprocal translocations: is the unbalanced mode at birth predictable? Hum Genet 91:228–232, 1993.

35. de la Chapelle A. Analytic review: nature and origin of males with XX sex chromosome. Am J Hum Genet 24:71–105, 1972.

36. Winderickx J, Battisti L, Hibiya Y, Motulsky AG, Deeb SS. Haplotype diversity in the human red and green opsin genes: evidence for frequnet sequence exchange in exon 3. Hum Mol Genet 2:1413–1421, 1993.

37. Madan K, Seabright M, Lindenbaum RH, Bobrow M. Paracentric inversions in man. (Review). J Med Genet 21:407–412, 1984.

38. Madan K. Paracentric inversions: a review. (Review). Hum Genet 96:503–515, 1995.
39. Anonymous. Pericentric inversions in man. A French collaborative study. Groupe de Cytogeneticiens Francais. (Review). Ann Genet 29:129–168, 1986.
40. Schroeder HW, Jr., Forbes S, Mack L, Davis S, Norwood TH. Recombination aneusomy of chromosome 5 associated with multiple severe congenital malformations. Clin Genet 30:285–292, 1986.
41. VanDyke DL, Weiss L, Logan M, Pai GS. The origin and behavior of two isodicentric bisatellited chromosomes. Am J Hum Genet 29:294–300, 1977.
42. Nowell PC, Hungerford DA. Chromosome studies on normal and leukemic human lymphocytes. J Natl Cancer Inst 25:85–109, 1960.
43. deKlein A, vanKessel AG, Grosveld G, Bartram CR, Hagemeijer A, Bootsma D, et al. A cellular oncogene is translocated to the Philadelphia chromosome in chronic myelocytic leukaemia. Nature 300:765–767, 1982.
44. Groffen J, Stephenson JR, Heisterkamp N, deKlein A, Bartram CR, Grosveld G. Philadelphia chromosomal breakpoints are clustered within a limited region, bcr, on chromosome 22. Cell 36:93–99, 1984.
45. Heisterkamp N, Stephenson JR, Groffen J, Hansen PF, deKlein A, Bartram CR, et al. Localization of the c-*abl* oncogene adjacent to a translocation break point in chronic myelocytic leukaemia. Nature 306:239–242, 1983.
46. Kaiser-McCaw B, Epstein AL, Kaplan HS, Hecht F. Chromosome 14 translocation in African and North American Burkitt's lymphoma. Int J Cancer 19:482–486, 1977.
47. Zech L, Haglund U, Nilsson K, Klein G. Characteristic chromosomal abnormalities in biopsies and lymphoid-cell lines from patients with Burkitt lymphomas. Int J Cancer 17:47–56, 1976.
48. Bernheim A, Berger R, Lenoir G. Cytogenetic studies on African Burkitt's lymphoma cell lines: t(2;8) and t(8;22) translocations. Cancer Genet Cytogenet 3:307–315, 1981.
49. Hamlyn PH, Rabbitts TH. Translocation joins c-myc and immunoglobulin gamma 1 genes in a Burkitt lymphoma revealing a third exon in the c-myc oncogene. Nature 304:135–139, 1983.
50. Rappold GA, Hameister H, Cremer T, Adolph S, Henglein B, Freese UK, et al. c-myc and immunoglobulin kappa light chain constant genes are on the 8q+ chromosome of three Burkitt lymphoma lines with t(2;8) translocations. EMBO J 3:2951–2955, 1984.
51. Hollis GF, Mitchell KF, Battey J, Potter H, Taub R, Lenoir GM, et al. A variant translocation places the lambda immunoglobulin genes 3' to the c-myc oncogene in Burkitt's lymphoma. Nature 307:752–755, 1984.
52. Gelman EP, Psallidopoulos MC, Paspas TS, Dalla-Favera R. Identification of reciprocal translocation sites within the c-myc oncogene and immunoglobulin mu locus in a Burkitt lymphoma. Nature 306:799–803, 1983.
53. Max EE, Seidman JG, Leder P. Sequences of five potential recombination sites encoded close to an immunoglobulin kappa constant region gene. Proc Natl Acad Sci USA 76:3450–3454, 1979.
54. Sakano H, Huppi K, Heinrich G, Tonegawa S. Sequences at the somatic recombination sites of immunoglobulin light-chain genes. Nature 280:288–294, 1979.
55. Bernard O, Hozumi N, Tonegawa S. Sequences of mouse immunoglobulin light chain genes before and after somatic changes. Cell 15:1133–1144, 1978.
56. Howard RO, Breg WR, Albert DM, Lesser RL. Retinoblastoma and chromosome abnormality. Partial deletion of the long arm of chromosome 13. Arch Ophthalmol 92:490–493, 1974.

57. Orye E, Delbeke MJ, Vandenabeele B. Retinoblastoma and long arm deletion of chromosome 13. Attempts to define the deleted segment. Clin Genet 5:457–464, 1974.

58. Riccardi VM, Sujansky E, Smith AC, Francke U. Chromosomal imbalance in the Aniridia-Wilms' tumor association: 11p interstitial deletion. Pediatrics 61:604–610, 1978.

59. Riccardi VM, Hittner HM, Francke U, Pippin S, Holmquist GP, Kretzer FL, et al. Partial triplication and deletion of 13q: study of a family presenting with bilateral retinoblastomas. Clin Genet 15:332–345, 1979.

60. Yunis JJ, Ramsay NK. Familial occurrence of the aniridia-Wilms tumor syndrome with deletion 11p13–14.1. J Pediatr 96:1027–1030, 1980.

61. Francke U, Kung F. Sporadic bilateral retinoblastoma and 13q- chromosomal deletion. Med Pediatr Oncol 2:379–385, 1976.

62. Pangalos C, Avramopoulos D, Blouin JL, Raoul O, deBlois MC, Prieur M, et al. Understanding the mechanism(s) of mosaic trisomy 21 by using DNA polymorphism analysis. Am J Hum Genet 54:473–481, 1994.

63. Antonarakis SE, Avramopoulos D, Blouin JL, Talbot CC, Jr, Schinzel AA. Mitotic errors in somatic cells cause trisomy 21 in about 4.5% of cases and are not associated with advanced maternal age. Nat Genet 3:146–150, 1993.

64. Hall JG. Genomic imprinting: review and relevance to human diseases. Am J Hum Genet 46:857–873, 1990.

65. Engel E. A new genetic concept: uniparental disomy and its potential effect, isodisomy. Am J Med Genet 6:137–143, 1980.

66. Pierre RV, Hoagland HC. 45,X cell lines in adult men: loss of Y chromosome, a normal aging phenomenon? Mayo Clin Proc 46:52–55, 1971.

67. Fitzgerald PH, McEwan CM. Total aneuploidy and age-related sex chromosome aneuploidy in cultured lymphocytes of normal men and women. Hum Genet 39:329–337, 1977.

68. Sandberg AA. The Chromosomes in Human Cancer and Leukemia. 2nd ed. New York: Elsevier, 1990.

69. Smith A, van Haaften-Day C, Russell P. Sequential cytogenetic studies in an ovarian cancer cell line. Cancer Genet Cytogenet 38:13–24, 1989.

70. Atkin NB. Modal DNA value and chromosome number in ovarian neoplasia. A clinical and histopathologic assessment. Cancer 27:1064–1073, 1971.

71. Spence JE, Perciaccante RG, Greig GM, Willard HF, Ledbetter DH, Hejtmancik JF, et al. Uniparental disomy as a mechanism for human genetic disease. Am J Hum Genet 42:217–226, 1988.

72. Voss R, Ben-Simon E, Avital A, Godfrey S, Zlotogora J, Dagan J, et al. Isodisomy of chromosome 7 in a patient with cystic fibrosis: could uniparental disomy be common in humans? Am J Hum Genet 45:373–380, 1989.

73. Nicholls RD, Knoll JH, Butler MG, Karam S, Lalande M. Genetic imprinting suggested by maternal heterodisomy in nondeletion Prader-Willi syndrome. Nature 342:281–285, 1989.

74. Gregory CA, Schwartz J, Kirkilionis AJ, Rudd N, Hamerton JL. Somatic recombination rather than uniparental disomy suggested as another mechanism by which genetic imprinting may play a role in the etiology of Prader-Willi syndrome. Hum Genet 88:42–48, 1991.

75. Hall JG. How imprinting is relevant to human disease. Dev Suppl:141–148, 1990.

76. Kalousek DK, Dill FJ, Pantzar T, McGillivray BC, Yong SL, Wilson RD. Confined chorionic mosaicism in prenatal diagnosis. Hum Genet 77:163–167, 1987.

77. Reik W, Brown KW, Slatter RE, Sartori P, Elliott M, Maher ER. Allelic methylation of H19 and IGF2 in the Beckwith-Wiedemann syndrome. Hum Mol Genet 3:1297–1301, 1994.

78. Weksberg R, Shen DR, Fei YL, Song QL, Squire J. Disruption of insulin-like growth factor 2 imprinting in Beckwith-Wiedmann syndrome. Nat Genet 5:143–150, 1993.

79. Welch TR, Beischel LS, Choi E, Balakrishnan K, Bishof NA. Uniparental isodisomy 6 associated with deficiency of the fourth component of complement. J Clin Invest 86:675–678, 1990.

80. Temple IK, Cockwell A, Hassold T, Pettay D, Jacobs P. Maternal uniparental disomy for chromosome 14. J Med Genet 28:511–514, 1991.

81. Wang JC, Passage MB, Yen PH, Shapiro LJ, Mohandas TK. Uniparental heterodisomy for chromosome 14 in a phenotypically abnormal familial balanced 13/14 Robertsonian translocation carrier. Am J Hum Genet 48:1069–1074, 1991.

82. Carpenter NJ, Say B, Barber ND. A homozygote for pericentric inversion of chromosome 4. J Med Genet 19 (6):469–471, 1982.

83. Kirkels VGHJ, Hustinx TWJ, Scheres JMJC. Habitual abortion and translocation (22q;22q): unexpected transmission from a mother to her phenotypically normal daughter. Clin Genet 18:456–461, 1980.

84. Palmer CG, Schwartz S, Hodes ME. Transmission of a balanced homologous t(22q;22q) translocation from mother to normal daughter. Clin Genet 17:418–422, 1980.

85. Knudson AG, Jr., Strong LC. Mutation and cancer: a model for Wilms' tumor of the kidney. J Natl Cancer Inst 48:313–324, 1972.

86. Knudson AG, Jr., Hethcote HW, Brown BW. Mutation and childhood cancer: a probabilistic model for the incidence of retinoblastoma. Proc Natl Acad Sci USA 72:5116–5120, 1975.

87. Knudson AG, Jr. Mutation and cancer: statistical study of retinoblastoma. Proc Natl Acad Sci USA 68:820–823, 1971.

88. Cavenee WK, Dryja TP, Phillips RA, Benedict WF, Godbout R, Gallie BL, et al. Expression of recessive alleles by chromosomal mechanisms in retinoblastoma. Nature 305:779–784, 1983.

89. Koufos A, Hansen MF, Lampkin BC, Workman ML, Copeland NG, Jenkins NA, et al. Loss of alleles at loci on human chromosome 11 during genesis of Wilms' tumour. Nature 309:170–171, 1984.

90. Friend SH, Horowitz JM, Gerber MR, Wang XF, Bogenmann E, Li FP, et al. Deletions of a DNA sequence in retinoblastomas and mesenchymal tumors: organization of the sequence and its encoded protein (published erratum appears in Proc Natl Acad Sci USA 1988 Apr;85(7):2234). Proc Natl Acad Sci USA 84:9059–9063, 1987.

91. Shah IC, Arlen M, Miller T. Osteogenic sarcoma developing after radiotherapy for retinoblastoma. Am Surg 40:485–490, 1974.

92. Yoneyama T, Greenlaw RH. Osteogenic sarcoma following radiotherapy for retinoblastoma. Radiology 93:1185–1186, 1969.

93. Toguchida J, Ishizaki K, Sasaki MS, Nakamura Y, Ikenaga M, Kato M, et al. Preferential mutation of paternally derived RB gene as the initial event in sporadic osteosarcoma. Nature 338:156–158, 1989.

94. Harbour JW, Lai SL, Whang-Peng J, Gazdar AF, Minna JD, Kaye FJ. Abnormalities in structure and expression of the human retinoblastoma gene in SCLC. Science 241:353–357, 1988.

95. Ponder B. Gene losses in human tumours. Nature 335:400–402, 1988.

96. Hansen MF, Cavenee WK. Retinoblastoma and the progression of tumor genetics. (Review). Trends Genet 4:125–128, 1988.

97. Schmickel RD. Contiguous gene syndromes: a component of recognizable syndromes. (Review). J Pediatr 109:231–241, 1986.

98. Francke U, Ochs HD, deMartinville B, Giacalone J, Lindgren V, Distéche C, et al. Minor Xp21 chromosome deletion in a male associated with XX expression of Duchenne muscular dystrophy, chronic granulomatous XX disease, retinitis pigmentosa,and McLeod syndrome. Am J Hum Genet 37:250–267, 1985.

99. Williams JD, Summitt RL, Martens PR, Kimbrell RA. Familial Down syndrome due to t(10;21) translocation: evidence that the Down phenotype is related to trisomy of a specific segment of chromosome 21. Am J Hum Genet 27:478–485, 1975.

100. Balfour B, Say B, Geffen WA, Morgan DG, Carpenter NJ, Munshi G. Down syndrome due to 21;21 translocation in a male twin. Clin Genet 16:383–386, 1979.

101. Richards BW. Mosaic mongolism. J Ment Def Res 13:66–83, 1969.

102. Taylor AI. Cell selection in vivo in normal/G trisomic mosaics. Nature 49:1028–1030, 1968.

103. Carr DH. Genetic basis of abortion. Adv Hum Genet 2:201–257, 1971.

104. de la Chapelle A, Schroder J, Kokkonen J. Cytogenetics of recurrent abortion or unsuccessful pregnancy. Int J Fertil 18:215–219, 1973.

105. Rosner F, Lee SL. Down syndrome and acute leukemia: myeloblastic or lymphoblastic? Am J Med 53:203–218, 1972.

106. Scully RE. Gonadoblastoma. A review of 74 cases. Cancer 25:1340–1356, 1970.

107. Bick D, Curry CJ, McGill JR, Schorderetk DF, Bux RC, Moore CM. Male infant with ichthyosis, Kallmann syndrome, chondrodysplasia punctata, and an Xp chromosome deletion. Am J Med Genet 33:100–107, 1989.

108. Brodeur GM, Dahl GV, Williams DL, Tipton RE, Kalwinsky DK. Transient leukemoid reaction and trisomy 21 mosaicism in a phenotypically normal newborn. Blood 55:691–693, 1980.

109. Weinberg AG, Schiller G, Windmiller J. Neonatal leukemoid reaction. An isolated manifestation of mosaic trisomy 21. Am J Dis Child 136:310–311, 1982.

110. Happle R. The lines of Blaschko: a developmental pattern visualizing functional X-chromosome mosaicism. Curr Probl Dermatol 17:5–18, 1987.

111. Happle R. Association of pigmentary anomalies with chromosomal and genetic mosaicism and chimerism. Am J Hum Genet 48:1013–1014, 1991.

112. Turleau C, Taillard F, Doussau-de-Bazignan M, Delepine N, Desbois JC, deGrouchy J. Hypomelanosis of Ito (incontinentia pigmenti achromians) and mosaicism for a microdeletion of 15q1. Hum Genet 74:185–187, 1986.

113. Donnai D, Read AP, McKeown C, Andrews T. Hypomelanosis of Ito: a manifestation of mosaicism or chimerism. J Med Genet 25:809–818, 1988.

114. Donnai D, McKeown C, Andrews T, Read AP. Diploid/triploid mixoploidy and hypomelanosis of Ito letter. Lancet 1:1443–1444, 1986.

115. Thomas IT, Frias JL, Cantu ES, Lafer CZ, Flannery DB, Graham JG, Jr. Association of pigmentary anomalies with chromosomal and genetic mosaicism and chimerism (see comments). (Review). Am J Hum Genet 45:193–205, 1989.

116. Happle R. Lethal genes surviving by mosaicism: a possible explanation for sporadic birth defects involving the skin. J Am Acad Dermatol 16:899–906, 1987.

117. Bijlsma JB, Wijffels J, Tegelaers W. C8 trisomy mosaicism syndrome. Helv Paediatr Acta 27:281–298, 1972.

118. Hunter AG, Clifford B, Cox DM. The characteristic physiognomy and tissue specific karyotype distribution in the Pallister-Killian syndrome. Clin Genet 28:47–53, 1985.

119. Kalousek DK, Dill FJ. Chromosomal mosaicism confined to the placenta in human conceptions. Science 221:665–667, 1983.

120. Kalousek DK, Barrett IJ, McGillivray BC. Placental mosaicism and intrauterine survival of trisomies 13 and 18. Am J Hum Genet 44:338–343, 1989.

121. Kalousek DK, Howard-Peebles PN, Olson SB, Barrett IJ, Dorfmann A, Black SH, et al. Confirmation of CVS mosaicism in term placentae and high-frequency of intrauterine growth-retardation association with confined placental mosaicism. Prenat Diagn 11:743–750, 1991.

122. Reindollar RH, Byrd JR, Hahn DH, Haseltine FP, McDonough PG. A cytogenetic and endocrinologic study of a set of monozygotic isokaryotic 45,X/46,XY twins discordant for phenotypic sex: mosaicism versus chimerism. Fertil Steril 47:626–633, 1987.

123. Gonsoulin W, Copeland KL, Carpenter RJ, Jr., Hughes MR, Elder FF. Fetal blood sampling demonstrating chimerism in monozygotic twins discordant for sex and tissue karyotype (46,XY and 45,X). Prenat Diagn 10:25–28, 1990.

124. Fujimoto A, Boelter WD, Sparkes RS, Lin MS, Battersby K. Monozygotic twins of discordant sex both with 45,X/46,X,idic(Y) mosaicism. Am J Med Genet 41:239–245, 1991.

125. Maddalena A, Sosnoski DM, Berry GT, Nussbaum RL. Mosaicism for an intragenic deletion in a boy with mild ornithine transcarbamylase deficiency. N Engl J Med 319:999–1003, 1988.

126. Weinstein LS, Shenker A, Gejman PV, Merino MJ, Friedman E, Spiegel AM. Activating mutations of the stimulatory G protein in the McCune-Albright syndrome. N Engl J Med 325:1688–1695, 1991.

127. Happle R. The McCune-Albright syndrome: a lethal gene surviving by mosaicism. Clin Genet 29:321–324, 1986.

128. Sheshadri R, Kutlaca RJ, Trainor K, Matthews C, Morley AA. Mutation rate of normal and malignant human lymphocytes. Cancer Res 47:407–409, 1987.

129. Langlois RG, Bigbee WL, Jensen RH. Measurements of the frequency of human erythrocytes with gene expression loss phenotypes at the glycophorin A locus. Hum Genet 74:353–362, 1986.

130. Crowe JF, Schull WJ, Neel JV. A Clinical, Pathological, and Genetic Study of Multiple Neurofibromatosis. Springfield, IL: Thomas, 1956.

131. Vogel F. Neue Untersuchungen zur Genetik des Retinoblastoms (Glioma retinae). Z Menschl Vererbun-Konstitu 34:205–236, 1957.

132. Baker TC. A quantitative and cytological study of germ cells in human ovaries. Proc R Soc Lond [Biol] 158:417–433, 1963.

133. Murphy EA, Cramer DW, Kryscio RJ, Brown CC, Pierce ER. Gonadal mosaicism and genetic counseling for X-linked recessive lethals. Am J Hum Genet 26:207–222, 1974.

134. Bradley TB, Wohl RC, Petz LD, Perkins HA, Reynolds RD. Possible gonadal mosaicism in a family with hemoglobin K:oln. Johns Hopkins Med J 146:236–240, 1980.

135. Hall JG, Dorst JP, Rotta J, McKusick VA. Gonadal mosaicism in pseudoachondroplasia. Am J Med Genet 28:143–151, 1987.

136. Bakker E, van-Broeckhoven C, Bonten EJ, van-de-Vooren MJ, Veenema H, Van-Hul W, et al. Germline mosaicism and Duchenne muscular dystrophy mutations. Nature 329:554–556, 1987.

137. Cohn DH, Starman BJ, Blumberg B, Byers PH. Recurrence of lethal osteogenesis imperfecta due to parental mosaicism for a dominant mutation in a human type I collagen gene (COL1A1). Am J Hum Genet 46:591–601, 1990.

138. Bakker E, Veenema H, den-Dunnen JT, van-Broeckhoven C, Grootscholten PM, Bonten EJ, et al. Germinal mosaicism increases the recurrence risk for 'new' Duchenne muscular dystrophy mutations. J Med Genet 26:553–559, 1989.

139. van Essen AJ, Abbs S, Baiget M, Bakker E, Boileau C, van Broeckhoven C, et al. Parental origin and germline mosaicism of deletions and duplications of the dystrophin gene: a European study. Hum Genet 88:249–257, 1992.

140. Wallis GA, Starman BJ, Zinn AB, Byers PH. Variable expression of osteogenesis imperfecta in a nuclear family is explained by somatic mosaicism for a lethal point mutation in the alpha 1(I) gene (COL1A1) of type I collagen in a parent. Am J Hum Genet 46:1034–1040, 1990.

141. Warburton D, Byrne J, Canki N. Chromosome anomalies and prenatal development: an atlas. Oxford: Oxford University Press, 1991.

142. Kalousek DK, Vekemans M. Confined placental mosaicism. J Med Genet 33:529–533, 1996.

143. Hsu LY, Yu M, Neu RL, Van Dyke DL, Benn PA, Bradshaw CL, et al. Rare trisomy mosaicism diagnosed in amniocytes, involving an autosome other than chromosomes 13, 18, 20, and 21: karyotype/phenotype correlations. Prenat Diagn 17:201–242, 1997.

144. Cohen MM, Jr. Wiedmann-Beckwith syndrome, imprinting, IGF2, and H19: implications for hemihyperplasia, associated neoplasms, and overgrowth. Am J Hum Genet 52:233–234, 1994.

145. Knoll JHM, Nicholls RD, Magenis RE, Graham JMJ, Lalande M, Latt SA. Angelman and Prader-Willi syndromes share a common chromosome 15 deletion but differ in parental origin of the deletion. Am J Med Genet 32:285–290, 1989.

146. Williams CA, Zori RT, Stone JW, Gray BA, Cantu ES, Ostrer H. Maternal origin of 15q11–13 deletions in Angelman syndrome suggests a role for genomic imprinting. Am J Med Genet 35:350–353, 1990.

147. Magenis RE, Toth-Fejel S, Allen LJ, Black M, Brown MG, Budden S, et al. Comparison of the 15q deletions in Prader-Willi and Angelman syndromes: specific regions, extent of deletions, parental origin, and clinical consequences. Am J Med Genet 35:333–349, 1990.

148. Alvardo M, Bocian M, Walker AP. Interstitial deletion of the long arm of chromosome 3: case report, review, and definition of a phenotype. Am J Med Genet 27:781–786, 1987.

149. Lejeune J, Lafourcade J, Vialatta J, Boeswillwald M, Seringe P, Turpin R. Trois cas de deletion partielle du bras court d'un chromosome 5. C R Acad Sci 257:3098–3102, 1963.

150. Cohen H, Walker H, Delhanty JDA, Lucas SB, Huehns ER. Congential spherorocytosis, B19 parvovirus infection, and inherited interstitial deletion of the short arm of chromosome 8. Br J Haematol 78:251–257, 1991.

151. Vincent C, Kalatzis V, Compain S, Leveillers J, Slim R, Graia F, et al. A proposed new contiguous gene syndrome on 8q consists of branchio-oto-renal(BOR) syndrome, Duane syndrome, a dominant form of hydrocephalus and trapeze aplasia, implications for mapping of the BOR gene. Hum Mol Genet 3:1859–1866, 1994.

152. Buhler EM, Malik NJ. The tricho-rhino-phalangeal syndrome(s): chromosome 8 long arm deletion: is there a shortest region of overlap between reported cases? TRPI and TRPII syndromes: are they separate entities? Am J Med Genet 19:113–119, 1984.

153. Andersen SR, Geertinger P, Larsen H-W, Mikkelsen M, Parving A, Vestermark S, et al. Anirida, cataract, and gonadoblastoma in a mentally retarded girl with deletion of chromosome 11: a clinicopathological case report. Ophthalmogica 176:171–177, 1978.

154. Phelan MC, Albiez KL, Flannery DB, Stevenson RE. The Prader-Willi syndrome and albinism in a black infant. Proc Greenwood Genet Center 7:27–29, 1988.

155. Robinson WP, Bottani A, Xie YG, Balakrishman J, Binkert F, Mächler M, et al. Molecular, cytogenetic, and clinical investigations of Prader-Willi syndrome patients. Am J Hum Genet 49:1219–1234, 1991.

156. Frynburg JS, Breg WR, Lindgren V. Diagnosis of Angelman syndrome in infants. Am J Med Genet 38:58–64, 1991.

157. Brook-Carter PT, Peral B, Ward CJ, Thompson P, Hughes J, Mahashwar MM, et al. Deletion of the TSC2 and PKD1 genes associated with severe infantile polycystic kidney disease: a contiguous gene syndrome. Nat Genet 8:328–332, 1994.

158. Wilkie AOM, Buckle VJ, Harris PC, Lamb J, Barton NJ, Reeders ST, et al. Clinical features and molecular analysis of the alpha-thalassemia/mental retardation syndromes. I. Cases due to deletion involving chromosome 16p13.3. Am J Hum Genet 46:1112–1126, 1990.

159. Dobyns WB, Stratton RF, Parke JT, Greenberg F, Nussbaum RL, Ledbetter DH. The Miller-Dieker syndrome: lissencephaly and monosomy 17p. J Pediatr 102:552–558, 1983.

160. Kline AD, White ME, Wapner R, Rojas K, Biesecker LG, Kamholz J, et al. Molecular analysis of 18q-syndrome—and correlation with phenotype. Am J Hum Genet 52:895–906, 1993.

161. Kelley RI, Zackai EH, Emanuel BS, Kistenmacher M, Greenberg F, Punnett HH. The association of the DiGeorge anomalad with parital monosomy of chromosome 22. J Pediatr 101:197–200, 1982.

162. de la Chapelle A, Herva R, Koisto M, Aula P. A deletion in chromosome 22 can cause DiGeorge syndrome. Hum Genet 57:253–256, 1981.

163. Scambler PJ, Kelly D, Lindsay E, Williamson R, Goldberg R, Shprintzen R, et al. Velo-cardio-facial syndrome associated with chromosome 22 deletions encompassing the DiGeorge locus. Lancet 339:1138–1139, 1992.

164. Renier WO, Nabben FAE, Hustinx TWJ, Veerkamp JH, Otten BJ, Ter Laak HJ, et al. Congenital adrenal hypoplasia, progressive muscular dystrophy, and severe mental retardation, in association with glycerol kinase deficiency, in male sibs. Clin Genet 24:243–251, 1983.

165. Collins FA, Murphy DL, Reiss AL, Sims KB, Lewis JG, Freund L, et al. Clinical, biochemical, and neuropsychiatric evaluation of a patient with a contiguous gene syndrome due to a microdeletion Xp11.3 including the Norrie disease locus and monoamine oxidase (MAOA and MAOB) genes. Am J Med Genet 42:127–134, 1992.

166. Aubourg PR, Sack GH, Jr., Moser H. Frequent alterations of visual pigment genes in adrenoleukodystrophy. Am J Hum Genet 42:408–413, 1988.

5

Sex Chromosome Transmission

Sex-linked transmission was the first exception to Mendel's rules to be identified in humans. In his work with sex-limited transmission, Wilson identified two key features.[1] First, males and females have different sex chromosome constitutions; thus, the mechanism of sex determination is genetically mediated and demonstrates a paternal origin effect. Second, X-linked traits in males demonstrate a maternal origin effect in their transmission. The third feature of the story, inactivation of one of the X chromosomes in the somatic cells of females, resulting in the equivalent expression of X-linked genes in the somatic cells of males and females, was identified half a century later by Mary Lyon.[2] Other features of sex chromosome transmission were discovered only in recent years.

BIOLOGY OF SEX CHROMOSOMES

Organization. Most of the genetic events that occur for autosomes are similar for sex chromosomes. During meiosis in oocyte precursors, the two X chromosomes pair and recombine throughout their length. During meiosis in spermatocyte precursors, the X and Y chromosomes pair at the tips of their short and long arms and undergo recombination.[3] The regions that are exchanged between the X and Y chromosomes are termed pseudoautosomal because alleles that are inherited within the region are not transmitted exclusively by males or females (Fig. 5.1).[4] Because genes within the pseudoautosomal region of the short arm are not subject to X inactivation and are, thus, expressed equally in males and females, they behave essentially as autosomal genes (Fig. 5.2). The distal long arms of the sex chromosomes also pair and recombine during meiosis in spermatocyte precursors, although no genes have been identified in this second pseudoautosomal region.[5]

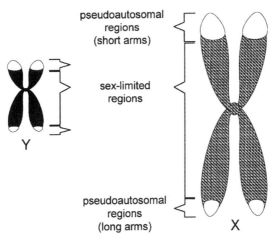

Figure 5.1. The pseudoautosomal regions are located at the ends of the short and long arms. These pair and recombine during male meiosis.

The other region of the sex chromosomes is termed *sex-limited* because genes within that region are linked to the sexual phenotype of the individual. Genes in the sex-limited region of the Y chromosome have a male-only pattern of transmission. Some of the genes that have been located in this region have functions that could occur only in males, such as testis determination and spermatogenesis.[6] Other genes that are located in the region have homologous copies on the X chromosome, even though recombination does not occur between these regions of the sex chromosomes.[7] As a result, these genes are unlikely to have a function exclusive to males.

X chromosome inactivation. As originally described by Mary Lyon in 1961, in individuals with two X chromosomes, one of the X chromosomes is randomly inactivated.[2] This phenomenon became known as the "Lyon hypothesis." Normally, one of the two X chromosomes is inactivated randomly in early embryos during the blastocyst stage of development.[8] The inactivation is thought to originate at a specific site on the long arm of the X chromosome (termed the *X chromosome inactivation center*) and to spread over the chromosome.[9] The inactivation is stable and is transmitted to the progeny cells.[10,11]

The process of X chromosome inactivation can skip over regions of the X chromosome affecting some genes, but not others.[12] In addition, the degree of inactivation at a given locus is variable, ranging from complete to none at all. Some of the loci that escape X chromosome inactivation have homologous genes on the sex-limited region of the Y chromosome. For example, in a given cell, the expression of one ZFX allele (a gene that has a Y chromosomal homologue, ZFY) has been found to be 30% of the expression of the other allele.[12] To date, it has not been demonstrated whether this level of expression is variable among individuals.

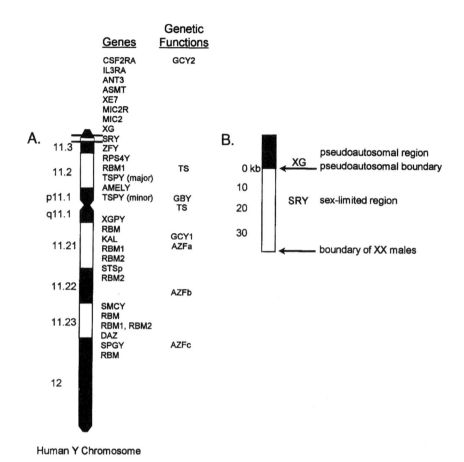

Human Y Chromosome

Figure 5.2. Maps of the human Y chromosome: (A) Detailed map showing genes and gene functions. The symbols for genes or genetic functions are as follows: CSF2RA, granulocyte-macrophage colony-stimulating factor receptor, α subunit; IL3RA, interleukin-3 receptor, α; ANT3, adenine nucleotide translocator-3; ASMT, acetylserotonin methyltransferase; XE7, pseudoautosomal gene XE7; MIC2R, MIC2-related gene; MIC2, surface antigen MIC2; XG, XG blood group system; SRY, sex-determining region Y; ZFY, zinc finger protein, Y-linked; RPS4Y, ribosomal protein S4, Y-linked; RBM1, RNA-binding motif protein; TSPY, testis-specific protein, Y-encoded; AMELY, amelogenin, Y-chromosomal; XGPY, XG blood group, pseudogene, Y-linked; KAL, Kallman syndrome; STSp, steroid sulfatase pseudogene; SMCY, selected mouse cDNA on Y; DAZ, deleted in azoospermia; SPGY, spermatogenesis gene on Y; TS, tooth size; GBY, gonadoblastoma; GCY, growth control on Y; AZF, azoospermia factor.

(B) Blowup of the pseudoautosomal boundary on the Y chromosome. The XG blood group straddles the boundary. The SRY gene starts 5 kb proximal to the boundary.

There are three molecular correlates of X chromosome inactivation. First, the inactive X chromosome replicates at a later time than the active chromosome.[13] A similar late pattern of replication occurs for the heterochromatic (dark-staining) regions of autosomes, where the genes are usually inactive and expressed only in a tissue-specific manner. Second, the XIST gene (for *X inactive-specific transcript*) is expressed from the *inactive* X chromosome.[14] This gene encodes an RNA which does not have an open reading frame nor is translated on polysomes.[15] Rather, the RNA transcript binds to sites on the inactive X chromosome.[16] Third, specific cytidine residues are methylated in genes on the inactive X chromosome.[17] It is unknown whether the methylation causes X chromosome inactivation or is a secondary phenomenon after the inactivation has occurred.

There are several factors that can influence the choice of X chromosome to inactivate. In the kangaroo and other marsupials, the paternally derived X chromosome is selectively inactivated in all somatic tissues of female animals.[18] By contrast, in humans and other eutherian mammals (specifically, mice and rats), selective inactivation of the paternally derived X chromosome occurs in the extraembryonic membranes in female animals.[19,20] This inactivation in eutherian mammals is selective but not absolute.[21,22] When there are two maternally derived X chromosomes, one of the X chromosomes is inactivated in the extraembryonic membranes.[23,24]

In some individuals, one X chromosome may be preferentially inactivated in a majority of cells.[25-28] Such skewing of X chromosome inactivation may occur by chance alone or may be the result of selection. In some cell types, skewed inactivation occurs because the expression of a mutant allele prevents cells from maturing along a developmental pathway. In cases of X-linked agammaglobulinemia, the B cells of heterozygous females express only the X chromosome that encodes the normal allele.[26] It is presumed that the absence of the gene product of the mutant allele prevents the precursors from maturing along the B cell pathway. By contrast in X-linked severe combined immunodeficiency syndrome, skewed X chromosome inactivation is observed in B cells as well as T cells.[29]

Selective inactivation of the normal (or untranslocated) X chromosome frequently occurs in individuals with balanced X-autosomal translocations.[30] In these cases, inactivation of the translocated X chromosome spreads to the autosomal segment. Monosomy for the autosomal regions is selected against either by suboptimal dosage of autosomal genes or by expression of deleterious alleles on the untranslocated autosome.

Positive selection may also occur for X chromosomes with deleterious alleles. For example, when cells from individuals with adrenomyeloneuropathy are grown in culture, the cells in which the mutant allele is expressed have a growth advantage over the normal cells; thus, although the phenotype of adrenoleukodystrophy is deleterious to the host, at a cellular level, the phenotype may be advantageous.[31]

If only a few precursor cells gave rise to a tissue or an organ and by chance these inactivated the same X chromosome, the pattern of X chromosome inactivation would appear to be skewed. This has been highlighted by differences in the patterns of X chromosome inactivation among the tissues of an individual and by discordance in the patterns of X chromosome inactivation between monozygotic twins.[32,33] As a result, one twin may have inherited a population of cells in which inactivation of the X chromosome bearing a mutant gene predominated, whereas the other twin inherited a population of cells in which inactivation of the normal X chromosome predominated. This can lead to discordant expression of X-linked phenotypes between the two twins in a pair.

X chromosome inactivation is not confined to females. Inactivation of X (and Y)-linked genes occurs during meiosis in male germ cells as the result of pairing and condensation of the sex chromosomes into a "sex vesicle."[34] The process of X chromosome inactivation is presumed to be similar to that in female somatic cells because the XIST gene is expressed in male germ cells.[35] Following meiosis, some X (and Y) linked genes are once again expressed.[36,37]

X chromosome reactivation. In oocytes, the X chromosome undergoes a process of reactivation.[38,39] As a result, gene expression in the oocyte does not appear to be subject to dosage compensation. For oogenesis to occur, expression of both alleles may be important for several loci.[40] Individuals with a single X chromosome or with a deletion of one of several different regions of the X chromosome have accelerated regression of the ovarian follicles and, thus, gonadal dysgenesis and infertility.

ABERRANT EXPRESSION OF X-LINKED GENES

Mendelian phenotypes. X-linked traits are characterized by absence of male-to-male transmission—that is, they may be transmitted from fathers to daughters or from mothers to daughters and sons. Depending on the number of copies of the gene that are required for expression, a given trait may be dominant or recessive.

Over 1,200 X-linked conditions have been described.[41] The presence of the hemizygous state in males makes it easier to map the genes for X-linked recessive conditions than the gene for other disorders. Some conditions have distinctive phenotypic features, whereas others are nonspecific. For example, over 40 different forms of X-linked mental retardation have been described. In some cases, the mental retardation is the only feature that has been discerned.[42] Originally, the X-linked nature of these conditions was inferred by the pattern of inheritance. More recently, the genes for these disorders have been localized to specific regions of the X chromosome using linkage to specific markers.[43]

Generally X-linked diseases are more likely to be expressed in males than in females, although there are a number of exceptions to this rule (Fig. 5.3). First, some conditions are dominant, so one copy of a gene is sufficient for the condition to be expressed. Second, affected females may be homozygous for the mutant allele. Third, they may be hemizygous with a 45,X karyotype. Finally, they may have skewed X chromosome inactivation in their cells, with the X

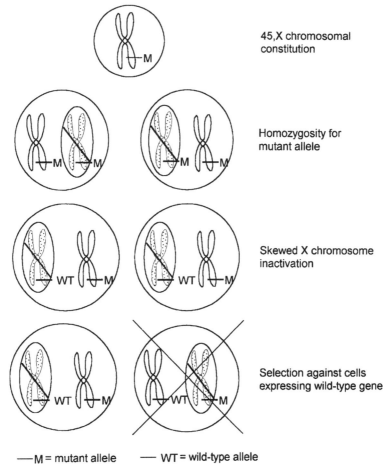

45,X chromosomal
constitution

Homozygosity for
mutant allele

Skewed X chromosome
inactivation

Selection against cells
expressing wild-type gene

—— M = mutant allele   —— WT = wild-type allele

Figure 5.3. Genetic factors that influence the expression of X-linked phenotypes in females. These include (A) 45,X chromosomal constitution, (B) homozygosity for mutant allele, (C) skewed X chromosome inactivation, and (D) selection against cells expressing the wild-type gene.

chromosome bearing the abnormal allele being preferentially expressed. As noted above, skewing may be a stochastic process or may be influenced by selection.

A priori, it is difficult to predict the pattern of inheritance that will be associated with a given mutation. Loss-of-function alleles have been observed for several X-linked dominant disorders (fragile X syndrome, adrenomyeloneuropathy, and hypophosphatemia rickets).[44–47] The severity of these conditions frequently correlates with skewed inactivation of the normal X chromosome; thus, the development of these conditions is explained by a fall in gene dosage below a critical level.[48–50]

The expression of X-linked recessive disorders in females is sometimes associated with X-autosomal translocations.[51] In these cases, inactivation of the translocated chromosome spreads into the autosomal region, leading to a functional monosomy for the autosomal genes. These cells are selected against and the normal X chromosome is preferentially inactivated in the surviving cells. If the translocation disrupts a gene, an X-linked phenotype is observed that corresponds to the disrupted locus. For example, many females with Duchenne muscular dystrophy and X-autosomal translocations have been identified.[52–57] The autosomal segments are variable in these translocations, but the breakpoint of the X chromosome always occurs within the dystrophin gene. The presence of site-specific X-autosomal translocations for other X-linked conditions identifies the map locations and has been useful for the positional cloning of the genes associated with these disorders (Table 5.1).

Male-lethal conditions. Some X-linked dominant conditions do not show Mendelian transmission because they are expressed only in females and usually as sporadic cases. The paucity of male cases is presumed to be the result of lethality during gestation. These conditions include incontinentia pigmenti,[58,59] Rett syndrome,[60] microphthalmia with linear skin defects (MLS),[61] and Aicardi syndrome.[62] Profound mental retardation is common to Rett, Aicardi, and MLS syndromes and sometimes occurs in incontinentia pigmenti syndrome. The occurrence of profound mental retardation explains the low genetic fitness and the apparent non-Mendelian transmission of these conditions. De novo X-autosomal translocations have been observed in occasional patients with some of these conditions, suggesting the map location of the genes (Table 5.2).

Aberrant chromosomal transmission. X-linked conditions may also be the result of aberrant chromosomal transmission. Among these conditions are 45,X, 47,XXX, and 47,XXY. Alteration of X chromosome dosage has a less profound effect on the viability of the host than autosomal dosage, for which most monosomies and trisomies are lethal. For the trisomies that involve an extra X chromosome, only one of the X chromosomes is active.[63] Nonetheless, individuals with these conditions have abnormal phenotypes. Individuals with a 47,XXX

Table 5.1. X-chromosomal Conditions Demonstrating Familial Transmission that Were Mapped in Females with X-Autosomal Translocations

Condition	X chromosome breakpoint
Duchenne muscular dystrophy[52–57]	Xp21
Aarskog syndrome[117]	Xp11
Norrie disease[118]	Xp11
Hypohidrotic ectodermal dysplasia[119,120]	Xq13.1
Menkes disease[121]	Xq13
Choroideremia[122]	Xq21.2
Lowe syndrome[123,124]	Xq25
Simpson-Golabi-Behmel syndrome[125]	Xq25-q27
Hunter syndrome[126]	Xq28
Torticollis, keloids, cryptorchidism, and renal dysplasia [127]	Xq28

Table 5.2. X-linked Conditions Associated with Male Lethality that Were Mapped in Females with X-autosomal Translocations

Condition	X chromosome breakpoint
Incontinentia pigmenti[128–131]	Xp11
Aicardi syndrome[132]	Xp22
Microphthalmia with linear skin defects[133–135]	Xp22
Rett syndrome[136,137]	Xp11 or Xp22

karyotype are more likely to have mental retardation and tall stature. Individuals with a 47,XXY karyotype have Klinefelter syndrome with relatively tall stature, a eunuchoid habitus, breast development, small testes with hyalinization of the testicular tubules, and infertility. These findings suggest that genes that are not subject to inactivation of the X chromosome affect the phenotype.[63]

45,X is the only monosomy that is viable with gestation, although it is estimated that about 90% of conceptuses with this condition are not carried to term. The condition is usually associated with gonadal dysgenesis and the Turner phenotype of webbed neck, shield chest, coarctation of the aorta, short stature, and renal malformations.[64] In 70–80% of infants with monosomy X, the single X chromosome is maternal in origin;[65] thus, they lack a paternally transmitted sex chromosome. There are two ways in which this could occur. First, the oocyte may be fertilized with a sperm that lacks a sex chromosome. Alternatively, there could be postzygotic loss of a paternally derived sex chromosome; however, as judged by cytogenetic and molecular analyses, postzygotic loss of a second sex chromosome accounts for only 10–15% of cases of Turner syndrome.

45,X monosomy is associated with gonadal dysgenesis, a process of partial or complete regression. The regression occurs when the genetic signals are not present for completing the differentiation process.[66] The association of gonadal dysgenesis with 45,X monosomy highlights the need for two structurally intact X chromosomes that are active in developing oocytes to prevent ovarian regression.[67] The regression that occurs in the absence of a second active X chromosome may be the result of subthreshold expression of certain genes required for ovarian development or of the expression of deleterious alleles that prevent the maturation process. This regression represents an acceleration of the process that occurs normally with oocytes. At 16 weeks of gestation, approximately 4 million oocytes are present in the ovaries of normal fetuses and those with 45,X monosomy. By the time of birth, fetuses with 45,X monosomy have virtually no oocytes.[68]

The steady state between ovarian follicle maintenance and follicle regression may be altered by the presence of sex chromosomal mosaicism in the gonad. Some individuals with 45,X/46,XX mosaicism have gonadal dysgenesis, whereas others do not.[69] The level of mosaicism in white cells or fibroblasts is not predictive of the level of mosaicism in the gonad. Some individuals for whom 45,X is the major cell line in peripheral blood make estrogens, go through puberty, and even have ovulatory cycles.[70,71]

Nonmosaic structural changes of the X chromosome have also been associated with gonadal dysgenesis.[72] These chromosomal variants suggest the locations of genes that are necessary for oocyte maturation. The most common structural variant associated with this phenotype is an isodicentric chromosome of the long arm of X.[73] Here, the long arm, the centromere, and part of the short arm are duplicated and the remainder of the short arm is deleted. Because genes on the short arm are necessary for viability, the isodicentric chromosome is preferentially inactivated in somatic cells. When X chromosome reactivation occurs in oocytes, suboptimal dosage for genes on the short arm of the X chromosome may lead to oocyte regression and gonadal dysgenesis. The alternative explanation, expression of deleterious recessive alleles on the normal X chromosome, appears less likely. The presence of specific X chromosome deletions in some women with gonadal dysgenesis provides further refinement of the map locations for such dosage-sensitive genes.[66,74,75]

Overexpression of X-linked genes. Duplication of the X chromosome also provides an indication for the location of dosage-sensitive genes. Several cases of 46,XY gonadal dysgenesis have been identified with duplications of the short arm of the X chromosome at Xp21-p22.[76–78] These individuals are likely to have increased expression for a gene or genes in this duplicated segment that suppressed the testis-determining effects of the Y chromosome. This gene ordinarily does not play a role in testis determination, because gonadal differentiation is not impaired in 46,XY males with deletion of this region.

Expression of genes from two active X chromosomes in the somatic cells of 46,XX females can also have deleterious effects. One way in which such overexpression occurs is as the result of a structural abnormality of the X chromosome that deletes the inactivation center. Ring chromosomes that have deletions of the X chromosome inactivation center are not subject to inactivation and have abnormal phenotypes that include mental retardation and other features.[79,80] These features are presumed to be the result of overexpression of X chromosomal loci in somatic cells. Such phenotypes are not observed in individuals with 47,XXX or 47,XXY phenotypes because the supernumerary X chromosomes are inactivated in the corresponding locations.

ABERRANT EXPRESSION OF Y-LINKED GENES

Y-chromosomal transmission meets Mendel's first rule of segregation of genes; however, there is no independent assortment of alleles. Furthermore, there is no recombination in the sex-limited region; thus, although Y-linked traits can be inferred on the basis of male-to-male transmission, they cannot be mapped using linkage analysis. Instead, the genes have been identified by phenotype–genotype correlation in individuals who have had aberrant transmission of Y-chromosomal fragments and by molecular mapping techniques. The major phenotypes that have been identified by aberrant Y-chromosomal transmission are sex reversal, infertility, Turner syndrome, gonadal tumor development, and increased stature.

Sex reversal. The first gene to be mapped to the Y chromosome causes the undifferentiated fetal gonad to differentiate into a testis. Based on cytogenetic analysis of males with deletions and translocations of the Y chromosome, this gene was mapped to the short arm of the Y chromosome.[81] The map position was further refined by analyzing 46,XX males and 46,XY females with gonadal dysgenesis. Unequal recombination involving the pseudoautosomal regions of the X and Y chromosomes can cause individuals with XX chromosomal constitutions to develop as males and individuals with XY chromosomal constitutions to develop as females (Fig. 5.4). If unequal pairing occurs between the two sex chromosomes followed by recombination, the X chromosome will contain a piece of the sex-specific region of the Y chromosome, including the testicular-determining factor (TDF), whereas the Y chromosome will lack TDF.[30,82] Aber-

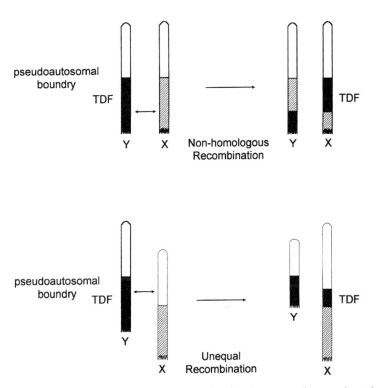

Figure 5.4. Genetic mechanisms leading to the development of XX males. These include nonhomologous recombination in the sex-limited regions of the X and Y chromosomes and unequal recombination between the sex-limited region on Y and the pseudoautosomal region on X.

rant recombination between sex chromosomes resulting in XX maleness is always de novo because the affected individuals are infertile.

In 1990, a gene called *sex-determining region Y* (SRY in humans, Sry in mice) was cloned from the 35-kb Y-chromosomal region of a 46,XX male with a small Y-to-X translocation.[83] A similar gene, Sry, was cloned from the sex-determining region of the Y chromosome of the mouse *Mus musculus molossinus*[84] and was found on the Y chromosomes of other eutherian mammals in which it was tested, including chimpanzee, rabbit, pig, horse, cow, and tiger.[83] Mutations in SRY are associated with gonadal dysgenesis in humans.[85–90] Human XX males can be mimicked in mice. Injection of the mouse Sry gene into XX mouse zygotes results in testicular differentiation.[91]

Infertility. Ordinarily a gene or set of genes on the long arm of the Y chromosome are required for normal sperm production to occur. Individuals who have interstitial deletions of the long arms of the Y chromosome may have infertility as their only phenotype.[92,93] These individuals have oligospermia, in which there is a decreased production of sperm, and azospermia, in which the production of sperm becomes arrested at an immature stage of development. In some cases, the deletions are too small to be observed microscopically.[94,95]

Deletion mapping on the Y chromosomes from individuals with oligo/azospermia has identified three regions that are necessary for normal spermatogenesis to occur.[94–98] Several genes that encode ribosomal binding proteins, including the RBM family of genes, DAZ1, and SPGY, have been mapped to these regions.[99–101]

Other genes inferred by phenotype–genotype correlation. One or more genes that prevent the development of the Turner phenotype are inferred to be present on the short arm of the Y chromosome because some individuals with deletions of the short arm have the Turner phenotype.[102–106] The distinguishing features appear to be both the length and the specific region of the Y-chromosomal segment that has been deleted in these individuals. Translocation of the short arm of the Y chromosome onto the X chromosome or an autosome results in male sexual differentiation in individuals with 45,X chromosomal constitutions.[81] Like 46,XX males, individuals with these phenotype have short stature and infertility. Unlike females with 45,X karyotypes, most do not have the Turner phenotype.[106] This suggests that the translocated segment includes a gene or genes that prevent development of the Turner phenotype. The presence of a gene in the pericentromeric region of the Y chromosome has been inferred to increase the risk for the development of gonadoblastoma because some individuals with gonadal dysgenesis and normal or structurally aberrant Y chromosomes develop tumors in their dysgenetic gonads.[107,108]

A dominant gene for stature may be present on the Y chromosome, because girls with 46,XY gonadal dysgenesis tend to be taller than girls with 46,XX gonadal dysgenesis.[109] By deletion mapping, this gene has been localized to proximal Yq.[110] Other Y-linked genes do not act in a dominant fashion in individuals with a 46,XX karyotype. This is based on the observation that 46,XX females who inherit a Y-autosomal translocation do not have readily identifiable phenotypic differences that can be ascribed to their Y chromosomes.[111]

Y-chromosomal genes identified by molecular mapping techniques. Several genes of unknown phenotypic significance were identified on the Y chromosome using molecular mapping techniques (Fig. 5.2). The TSPY gene has 20–40 copies on Yp.[112] This gene encodes a 33-kD phosphoprotein that is expressed in spermatogonia, testicular carcinoma in situ, and some seminomas. TSPY is homologous to the proto-oncogene SET.[101] PRKY (for *protein kinase Y chromosome*) is also located on Yp.[113] This gene was located on the Y chromosome based on its homology with the X-linked gene, PRKX. The X- and Y-linked genes act as hotspots for illegitimate recombination between the X and Y chromosomes in forming X-Y translocations.[47,113]

The gene for the XG blood group has two copies on the Y chromosome. The Y homologue of the XG blood group maps to long arm and is transcribed.[114] By contrast, the gene for the XG blood group straddles the pseudoautosomal boundary. Two exons that are necessary for expressing an intact gene product are not present in the sex-specific region of the Y chromosome.[115,116]

CONSEQUENCES OF SEX CHROMOSOME TRANSMISSION

Sex chromosome transmission causes deviations from Mendelian genetics in several ways. It causes parent-of-origin effects and leads to sex-limited expression of genetic traits. By its nature, X chromosome inactivation is a cause of variable expressivity of genetic traits among females within a family. Genes on both sex chromosomes play a crucial role in sexual differentiation and in germ cell maturation.

Sex chromosome transmission was the first parent-of-origin effect to be identified. Others followed on its heels. By the mid 1930s it was suspected that cytoplasmic (maternal-only) transmission might occur for certain traits. Subsequently, cytoplasmic transmission was shown to be mediated by the mitochondria.

REFERENCES

1. Wilson EB. The sex chromosomes. Arch Mikrosk Anat Enwicklungsmech 77:249–271, 1911.
2. Lyon MF. Gene action in the X-chromosome of the mouse (Mus musculus). Nature 190:372–373, 1961.
3. Hulten M, Lindsten J, Ming PM, Fracaro M. The XY bivalent in human male meiosis. Ann Hum Genet 30:119–123, 1966.
4. Simmler M, Rouyer F, Vergnaud G, Nystrom-Lahti M, Ngo KY, de la Chapelle A, et al. Pseudoautosomal DNA sequences in the pairing region of the human sex chromosomes. Nature 317:692–697, 1985.

5. Freije D, Helms C, Watson MS, Donis-Keller H. Identification of a second pseudo-autosomal region near the Xq and Yq telomeres. Science 258:1784–1787, 1992.

6. Affara NA, Lau YF, Briggs H, Davey P, Jones MH, Kwaja O, et al. Report and abstracts of the FIRST International Workshop on Y Chromosome Mapping 1994. Cambrige, England, April 2–5, 1994. Cytogenet Cell Genet 67:359–402, 1994.

7. Page DC, Mosher R, Simpson EM, Fisher EM, Mardon G, Pollack J, et al. The sex-determining region of the human Y chromosome encodes a finger protein. Cell 51:1091–1104, 1987.

8. Epstein CJ, Smith S, Travis B, Tucker G. Both X chromosomes function before visible X-chromosome inactivation in female mouse embryos. Nature 274:500–503, 1978.

9. Russell LB. Mammalian X-chromosome action: inactivation limited in spread and in region of origin. Science 133:1795–803, 1963.

10. Gartler SM, Riggs AD. Mammalian X-chromosome inactivation. Annu Rev Genet 17:155–190, 1983.

11. Gartler SM, Dyer KA, Goldman MA. Mammalian X chromosome inactivation. Mol Genet Med 2:121–160, 1992.

12. Schneider-Gadicke A, Beer-Romero P, Brown LG, Nussbaum R, Page DC. ZFX has a gene structure similar to ZFY, the putative human sex determinant, and escapes X inactivation. Cell 57:1247–1258, 1989.

13. Taylor JH. Asynchronous duplication of chromosomes in cultured cells of Chinese hamster. J Biophys Biochem Cytol 7:455–464, 1960.

14. Brown CJ, Ballabio A, Rupert JL, Lafreniere RG, Grompe M. A gene from the region of the human X inactivation center is expressed exclusively from the inactive X chromosome. Nature 349:38–44, 1991.

15. Brown CJ, Hendrich BD, Rupert JL, Lafreniere RG, Xing Y, Lawrence J, et al. The human XIST gene: analysis of a 17 kb inactive X-specific RNA that contains conserved repeats and is highly localized within the nucleus. Cell 71:527–542, 1992.

16. Clemson CM, McNeil JA, Willard HF, Lawrence JB. XIST RNA paints the inactive X chromosome at interphase: evidence for a novel RNA involved in nuclear/chromosome structure. J Cell Biol 132:259–275, 1996.

17. Riggs AD. X inactivation, differentiation and DNA methylation. Cytogenet Cell Genet 14:9–25, 1975.

18. Sharman GB. Late DNA replication in the paternally derived X chromosome of the female kangaroo. Nature 230:231–232, 1971.

19. Takagi N, Wake N, Sasaki M. Cytologic evidence for preferential inactivation of the paternally derived X chromosome in XX mouse blastocysts. Cytogenet Cell Genet 20:240–248, 1978.

20. Ropers HH, Wolff G, Hitzeroth HW. Preferential X inactivation in human placenta membranes: is the paternal X inactive in early embryonicdevelopment of female mammals? Hum Genet 43:265–273, 1978.

21. Cattanach BM. Control of chromosome inactivation. Annu Rev Genet 9:1–18, 1975.

22. Papaioannou VE, West JD. Relationship between the parental origin of the X chromosomes, embryonic cell lineage and X chromosome expression in mice. Genet Res 37:183–197, 1981.

23. Kaufman MH, Guc-Cabrilo M, Lyon MF. X chromosome inactivation in diploid parthenogenetic mouse embryos. Nature 271:547–549, 1978.

24. Rastan S, Kaufman MH, Handyside AH, Lyon MF. X chromosome inactivation in extraembryonic membranes of diploid parthenogenetic mouse embryos demonstrated by differential staining. Nature 288:172–173, 1980.

25. Allen RC, Nachtman RG, Rosenblatt HM, Belmont JW. Application of carrier testing to genetic counseling for X-linked agammaglobulinemia. Am J Hum Genet 54:25–35, 1994.

26. Conley ME, Brown P, Pickard AR, Buckley RH, Miller DS, Raskind WH, et al. Expression of the gene defect in x-linked agammaglobulinemia. N Engl J Med 315:564–567, 1986.

27. Fialkow PJ. Primordial cell pool size and lineage relationships of five human cell types. Am J Hum Genet 37:39–48, 1973.

28. Fey MF, Liechti-Gallati S, von Rohr A, Borisch B, Theilkas L, Schneider V, et al. Clonality and X-inactivation patterns in hematopoietic cell populations detected by the highly informative M27 beta DNA Probe. Blood 83:931–938, 1994.

29. Puck JM, Nussbaum RL, Conley ML. Carrier detection in X-linked svere combined immunodeficiency based on patterns of X chromosome inactivation. J Clin Invest 79:1395–1400, 1987.

30. Zabel BU, Baumann WA, Pirntke W, Gerhard-Ratschow K. X-inactivation pattern in three cases of X/autosome translocation. Am J Med Genet 1:309–317, 1978.

31. Migeon BR, Moser HW, Moser AB, Axelman J, Sillence D, Norum RA. Adrenoleukodystrophy: evidence for X linkage, inactivation, and selection favoring the mutant allele in heterozygous cells. Proc Natl Acad Sci USA 78:5066–5970, 1981.

32. Gale RE, Wheadon H, Boulos P, Linch DC. Tissue-specificity of X-chromosome inactivation patterns. Blood 83:2899–2905, 1994.

33. Richards CS, Watkins SC, Hoffman EP, Schneider NR, Milsark IW, Katz KS, et al. Skewed X inactivation in a female MZ twin results in Duchenne muscular dystrophy. Am J Hum Genet 46:672–681, 1990.

34. Solari AJ. The behavior of the XY pair in mammals. Int Rev Cytol 38:273–317, 1974.

35. Richler C, Soreq H, Wahrman J. X inactivation in mammalian testis is correlated with inactive X-specific transcription. Nat Genet 2:192–195, 1992.

36. Hendriksen FJ, Hoogerbrugge JW, Themmen AP, Koken MH, Hoeijmakers JH, Oostra BA, et al. Postmeiotic transcritpion of X and Y chromosomal genes during spermatogenesis in the mouse. Dev Biol 170:730–733, 1995.

37. Nagamine CM, Chan K, Hake LE, Lau YF. The two candidate testis-determining Y genes (Zfy-1 and Zfy-2) are differentially expressed in fetal and adult mosue tissues. Genes Dev 4:63–74, 1990.

38. Kratzer PG, Chapman VM. X chromosome reactivation in oocytes of Mus caroli. Proc Natl Acad Sci USA 78:3093–3097, 1981.

39. Monk M, McLaren A. X-chromosome inactivation in foetal germ cells of the mouse. J Embryol Exp Morph 63:75–84, 1981.

40. Ostrer H. Sex determination. In: Adashi EY, Rock JA, Rosenwaks Z, editors. Reproductive Endocrinology: Surgery and Technology. New York: Raven Press, 1995:41–58.

41. McKusick VA. Mendelian Inheritance in Man. 8th ed. Baltimore: Johns Hopkins University Press, 1988.

42. Spano LM, Opitz JM. Bibliography on X-linked mental retardation, the fragile X and related subjects IV. Am J Med Genet 30 (1–2):31–60, 1988.

43. Neri G, Chiurazzi P, Arena F, Lubs HA, Glass IA. XLMR genes: update 1992. Am J Med Genet 43:373–382, 1992.

44. Pieretti M, Zhang FP, Fu YH, Warren ST, Oostra BA, Caskey CT, et al. Absence of expression of the FMR-1 gene in fragile X syndrome. Cell 66:817–822, 1991.

45. Mosser J, Douar A-M, Sarde C-O, Kioschis P, Feil R, Moser H, et al. Putative

X-linked adrenoleukodystrophy gene shares unexpected homology with ABC transporters. Nature 361:726–730, 1993.

46. Mosser J, Lutz Y, Stoeckel ME, Sarde CO, Kretz C, Douar AM, et al. The gene responsible for adrenoleukodystrophy encodes a peroxisomal membrane protein. Hum Mol Genet 3:265–271, 1994.

47. Anonymous. HYP Consortium: a gene (HYP) with homologies to endopeptidases is mutated in patients with X-linked hypophosphatemic rickets. Nat Genet 11:130–136, 1995.

48. Watkiss E, Webb T, Bundey S. Is skewed X inactivation responsible for symptoms in female carriers for adrenoleucodystrophy? J Med Genet 30:651–654, 1993.

49. Kirschgessner CU, Warren ST, Willard HF. X inactivation of the FMR1 fragile X mental retardation gene. J Med Genet 32:925–929, 1995.

50. Rousseau F, Heitz D, Tarleton J, MacPherson J, Malmgren H, Dahl N, et al. A multicenter study on genotype-phenotype correlations in the fragile X syndrome, using direct diagnosis with probe StB12.3: the first 2,253 cases. Am J Hum Genet 55:225–237, 1994.

51. Schmidt M, Du Sart D. Functional disomies of the X chromosome influence the cell selection and hence the X inactivation pattern in females with balanced X-autosome translocations: a review of 122 cases. Am J Med Genet 42:161–169, 1992.

52. Lidenbaum RH, Clarke G, Patel C, Moncrieff M, Hughes JT. Muscular dystrophy in an X;1 translocation female suggests that Duchenne locus is on X chromosome short arm. J Med Genet 16:389–392, 1979.

53. Worton RG, Duff C, Sylvester JE, Schmickel RD, Willard HF. Duchenne muscular dystrophy involving translocation of the DMD gene next to ribosomal RNA genes. Science 224:1447–1449, 1984.

54. Emanuel BS, Zackai EH, Tucker SH. Further evidence for Xp21 location of Duchenne muscular dystrophy (DMD) locus: X;9 translocation in a female with DMD. J Med Genet 20:461–463, 1983.

55. Zatz M, Vianna-Morgante AM, Campos P, Diament AJ. Translocation (X;6) in a female with Duchenne muscular dystrophy: implications for the localisation of the DMD locus. J Med Genet 18:442–447, 1981.

56. Jacobs PA, Hunt PA, Mayer M, Bart RD. Duchenne muscular dystrophy (DMD) in a female with an X/autosome translocation: further evidence that the DMD locus is at Xp21. Am J Hum Genet 33:513–518, 1981.

57. Greenstein RM, Reardon MP, Chan TS, Middleton AB, Mulivor RA, Greene AE, et al. An (X;11) translocation in a girl with Duchenne muscular dystrophy. Cytogenet Cell Genet 27:268, 1980.

58. Pfeiffer RA. Zur Frage der Vererbung der Incontinentia pigmenti Bloch-Siemens. Z Menschl Vererb Konstitutionsl 35:469–493, 1960.

59. Lenz W. Zur Genetik der Incontinentia pigmenti. Ann Paediat 196:149–165, 1961.

60. Hagberg B, Aicardi J, Dias K, Ramos O. A progressive syndrome of autism, dementia, ataxia, and loss of purposeful hand use in girls: Rett's syndrome: report of 35 cases. Ann Neurol 14:471–479, 1983.

61. Lindsay EA, Grillo A, Ferrero GB, Roth EJ, Magenis E, Grompe M, et al. Microphthalmia with linear skin defects (MLS) syndrome: clinical, cytogenetic, and molecular characterization. Am J Med Genet 49:229–234, 1994.

62. Aicardi J, Chevrie JJ, Rousselie F. Le syndrome spasnes en flexion, agenesic calleluse, anomalies chorio-retiniennes. Arch Fr Pediatr 26:1103–1120, 1969.

63. Lyon MF. Sex chromatin and gene action in the mammalian X-chromosome. Am J Hum Genet 14:135–148, 1962.

64. Hall JG, Gilchrist DM. Turner syndrome and its variants. Pediatr Clin North Am 37:1421–1440, 1990.

65. Mathur A, Stekol L, Schatz D, MacLaren NK, Scott ML, Lippe B. The parental origin of the single X chromosome in Turner syndrome: lack of correlation with parental age or clinical phenotype. Am J Hum Genet 48:682–686, 1991.

66. Simpson JL. Abnormal sexual differentiation in humans. Annu Rev Genet 16:193–224, 1982.

67. Monk M. The X chromosome in development in mouse and man. J Inherit Metab Dis 15:499–513, 1992.

68. Singh RP, Carr DH. The anatomy and histology of XO human embryos and fetuses. Anat Rec 155:369–383, 1966.

69. Kaplowitz PB, Bodurtha J, Brown J, Spence JE. Monozygotic twins discordant for Ullrich-Turner syndrome. Am J Med Genet 41:78–82, 1991.

70. McCorquodale MM, Bowdle FC. Two pregnancies and the loss of the 46,XX cell line in a 45,X/46,XX Turner mosaic patient. Fertil Steril 43:229–233, 1985.

71. Ayuso MC, Bello MJ, Benitez J, Sanchez-Cascos A, Mendoza G. Two fertile Turner women in a family. Clin Genet 26:591–596, 1984.

72. Simpson JL. Disorders of gonads and internal reproductive organs. In: Emery AEH, Rimoin DL, editors. Principles and Practice of Medical Genetics. 2nd ed. Edinburgh: Churchill Livingstone, 1990:1593–1617.

73. Therman E, Patau K. Abnormal X chromosomes in man: origin, behavior and effects. Humangenetik 25:1–16, 1974.

74. Simpson JL. Genes, chromosomes, and reproductive failure. Fertil Steril 33:107–116, 1980.

75. Krauss CM, Turksoy N, Atkins L, McLaughlin C, Brown LG, Page DC. Familial premature ovarian failure due to an interstitial deletion of the long arm of the X chromosome. N Engl J Med 317:125–131, 1987.

76. Bernstein R, Koo GC, Wachtel SS. Abnormality of the X chromosome in human 46,XY female siblings with dysgenic ovaries. Science 207:768–769, 1980.

77. Scherer G, Schempp W, Baccichetti C, Lenzini E, Bricarelli FD, Carbone LD et al. Duplications of an Xp segment that includes the ZFX locus causes sex reversal in men. Hum Genet 81:291–294, 1989.

78. Ogata T, Hawkins JR, Taylor A, Matsuo N, Hata J, Goodfellow PN. Sex reversal in a child with a 46,X,Yp+ karyotype: support for the existence of a gene(s), located in distal Xp, involved in testis formation. J Med Genet 29:226–230, 1992.

79. Wolff DJ, Brown CJ, Schwartz S, Duncan AM, Surti U, Willard HF. Small marker X chromosomes lack the X inactivation center: implications for karyotyping/phenotype correlations. Am J Hum Genet 55:87–95, 1994.

80. Migeon BR, Luo S, Stasiowski BA, Jani M, Axelman J, Van Dyke DL, et al. Deficient transcription of XIST from tiny ring X chromosomes in females with severe phenotypes. Proc Natl Acad Sci USA 90:12025–12029, 1993.

81. de la Chapelle A. Genetic and molecular studies on 46,XX and 45,X males. Cold Spring Harb Symp Quant Biol 51 Pt 1:249–255, 1986.

82. Petit C, de la Chapelle A, Levilliers J, Castillo S, Noel B, Weissenbach J. An abnormal terminal X-Y interchange accounts for most but not all cases of human XX males. Cell 49:595–602, 1987.

83. Sinclair AH, Berta P, Palmer MS, Hawkins JR, Griffiths BL, Smith MJ, et al. A gene from the human sex-determining region encodes a protein with homology to a conserved DNA-binding motif. Nature 346:240–244, 1990.

84. Gubbay J, Collignon J, Koopman P, Capel B, Economou A, Munsterberg A, et al.

A gene mapping to the sex-determining region of the mouse Y chromosome is a member of a novel family of embryonically expressed genes. Nature 346:245–250, 1990.

85. Berta P, Hawkins JR, Sinclair AH, Taylor A, Griffiths BL, Goodfellow PN, et al. Genetic evidence equating SRY and the testis-determining factor. Nature 348:448–450, 1990.

86. Jager RJ, Anvret M, Hall K, Scherer G. A human XY female with a frame shift mutation in the candidate testis-determining gene SRY. Nature 348:452–454, 1990.

87. Hawkins JR, Taylor A, Goodfellow PN, Migeon CJ, Smith KD, Berkovitz GD. Evidence for increased prevalence of SRY mutations in XY females with complete rather than partial gonadal dysgenesis. Am J Hum Genet 51:979–984, 1992.

88. Berkovitz GD, Fechner PY, Marcantonio SM, Bland G, Stetten G, Goodfellow PN, et al. The role of the sex-determining region of the Y chromosome (SRY) in the etiology of 46,XX true hermaphroditism. Hum Genet 88:411–416, 1992.

89. Muller J, Schwartz M, Skakkebaek NE. Analysis of the sex-determining region of the Y chromosome (SRY) in sex reversed patients: point-mutation in SRY causing sex-reversion in a 46,XY female. J Clin Endocrinol Metab 75:331–333, 1992.

90. McElreavey KD, Vilain E, Boucekkine C, Vidaud M, Jaubert F, Richaud F, et al. XY sex reversal associated with a nonsense mutation in SRY. Genomics 13:838–840, 1992.

91. Koopman P, Gubbay J, Vivian N, Goodfellow P, Lovell-Badge R. Male development of chromosomally female mice transgenic for Sry. Nature 351:117–121, 1991.

92. Tiepolo L, Zuffardi O. Localization of factors controlling spermatogenesis in the nonfluorescent portion of the hyman Y chromosome long arm. Hum Genet 34:119–124, 1976.

93. Chandley AC, Gosden JR, Hargreave TB, Spowart G, Speed RM, McBeath S. Deleted Yq in the sterile son of a man with a satellited Y chromosome (Yqs). J Med Genet 26:145–153, 1989.

94. Ma K, Sharkey A, Kirsch S, Vogt P, Keil R, Hargreave T, et al. Towards the molecular localisation of the AZF locus: Mapping of microdeletions in azoospermic men within 14 subintervals of interval 6 of the human Y chromosome. Hum Mol Genet 1:29–33, 1992.

95. Vogt P, Chandley AC, Hargreave TB, Keil R, Ma K, Sharkey A. Microdeletions in interval 6 of the Y chromosome of males with idiopathic sterility point to disruption of AZF, a human spermatogenesis gene. Hum Genet 89:491–496, 1992.

96. Henegariu O, Hirschmann P, Kilian P, Kirsch S, Lengauer C, Maiwald R, et al. Rapid screening of the Y chromosome in idiopatic sterile men, diagnstic for deletion in AZF, a genetic Y-factor expressed during spermatogenesis. Andrologia 26:97–106, 1994.

97. Kobayashi K, Mizuno K, Hida A, Kornaki R, Tomita K, Matsushita I, et al. PCR analysis of the Y chromosome long arm, in azospermic patients: evidence for a second locus required for spermatogenesis. Hum Mol Genet 3:1965–1967, 1994.

98. Kobayashi K, Mizuno K, Hida A, Komaki R, Tomita K, Matsushita I, et al. PCR analysis of the Y chromosome long arm in azospermic patients: evidence for a second locus required for spermatogenesis. Hum Mol Genet 3:1965–1967, 1994.

99. Ma K, Inglis JD, Sharkey A, Bickmore WA, Hill RE, Prosser EJ, et al. A Y chromosome gene family with RNA-binding protein homology: candidates for the azoospermia factor AZF controlling human spermatogenesis. Cell 75:1287–1295, 1993.

100. Reijo R, Lee T-Y, Salo P, Alagappan R, Brown LG, Rosenberg M, et al. Diverse spermatogenic defects in humans caused by Y chromosome deletions encompassing a novel RNA-binding protein gene. Nat Genet 10:383–393, 1995.

101. Affara N, Nischop C, Brown W, Cooke H, Davey P, Ellis N, et al. Report of the second international workshop on Y chromosome mapping 1995. Cytogenet Cell Genet 73:33–76, 1996.

102. Blagowidow N, Page DC, Huff D, Mennuti MT. Ullrich-Turner syndrome in an XY female fetus with deletion of the sex-determining portion of the Y chromosome. Am J Med Genet 34:159–162, 1989.

103. Ogata T, Tyler-Smith C, Purvis-Smith S, Turner G. Chromosomal localization of a gene(s) for Turner stigmata on Yp. J Med Genet 30:918–922, 1993.

104. Barbaux S, Vilain E, Raoul O, Gilgenkrantz S, Jeandidier E, Chadenas D, et al. Proximal deletions of the long arm of the Y chromosome suggest a critical region associated with a specific subset of characteristic Turner stigmata. Hum Mol Genet 4:1565–1568, 1995.

105. Calzolari E, Patracchini P, Palazzi P, Aiollo V, Ferlini A, Trasforini G, et al. Characterization of a deleted Y chromosome in a male with Turner stigmata. Clin Genet 43:16–22, 1993.

106. Weil D, Portnoi MF, Levilliers J, Wang I, Mathieu M, Taillemite JL, et al. A 45,X male with an X-Y translocation—implications for the genes responsbile for Turner syndrome and X-linked chondroplasia punctata. Hum Mol Genet 2:1851–1856, 1993.

107. Verp MS, Simpson JL. Abnormal sexual differentiation and neoplasia. Cancer Genet 25:191–218, 1987.

108. Tsuchiya K, Reijo R, Page DC, Disteche CM. Gonadoblastoma: molecular definition of the susceptibility region on the Y chromosome. Am J Hum Genet 57:1400–1407, 1995.

109. Ogata T, Matsuo N. Comparison of adult height between patients with XX and XY gonadal dysgenesis: support for a Y specific growth gene(s). J Med Genet 29:539–541, 1992.

110. Ogata T, Tomita K, Hida A, Matsuo N, Nakahori Y, Nakagome Y. Chromosomal localisation of a Y specific growth gene(s). J Med Genet 32:572–575, 1995.

111. Ostrer H, Henderson AL, Stringer LC. Characterization of Y chromosomal deoxyribonucleic acid fragments and translocations by Southern blot analysis. J Pediatr 111:678–683, 1987.

112. Arnemann J, Epplen J, Cooke H, Sauermann U, Engel W, Schmidtke J. A human Y-chromosomal DNA sequence expessed in testicular tissue. Nucleic Acids Res 15:8713–8724, 1987.

113. Klink A, Schiebel K, Winkelmann M, Rao E, Horstmeke B, Ludecke H-J, et al. The human protein kinase gene PKX1 on Xp22.3 displays Xp/Yp homology and is a site of chromosomal instability. Hum Mol Genet 4:869–878, 1995.

114. Ellis N, Ye T, Patton S, Weller P. PBDX, an MIC2-related gene that spans the pseudoautosomal boundary on Xp, and PBDY, a Y-specific duplication of PBDX, on Yq. Cytogenet Cell Genet 67:390–391, 1994.

115. Ellis NA, Tippett P, Petty A, Reid M, Weller PA, Ye T-Z, et al. PBDX is the XG blood group gene. Nat Genet 8:285–290, 1994.

116. Weller PA, Critcher R, Goodfellow PN, German J, Ellis NA. The human Y-chromosome homolog of XG—transcription of a naturally trunacted gene. Hum Mol Genet 2:1853–1856, 1995.

117. Glover TW, Verga V, Rafael J, Varcroft C, Gorski JL, Bawle EV, et al. Transloca-

tion breakpoint in Aarskog syndrome maps to Xp11.21 between ALAS2 and DXS323. Hum Mol Genet 2:1717–1718, 1993.

118. Ohba N, Yamashita T. Primary vitreoretinal dysplasia resembling Norrie's disease in a female: association with X autosomal chromosomal translocation. Br J Ophthalmol 70:64–71, 1986.

119. Zonana J, Clarke A, Sarfarazi M, Thomas NST, Roberts K, Marymee K, et al. X-linked hypohydrotic ectodermal dysplasia: localization within the region Xq11–21.1 by linkage analysis and implications for carrier detection and prenatal diagnosis. Am J Hum Genet 43:75–85, 1988.

120. Turleau C, Niaudet P, Cabanis M-O, Plessis G, Cau D, de Grouchy J. X-linked hypohidrotic ectodermal dysplasia and t(X;12) in a female. Clin Genet 35:462–466, 1989.

121. Kapur S, Higgins JV, Delp K, Rogers B. Menkes syndrome in a girl with X-autosome translocation. Am J Med Genet 26:503–510, 1987.

122. Siu VM, Gonder JR, Jung JH, Sergovich FR, Flintoff WF. Choroideremia associated with an X-autosomal translocation. Hum Genet 84:459–464, 1990.

123. Hodgson SV, Heckmatt JZ, Hughes E, Crolla JA, Dubowitz V, Bobrow M. A balanced de novo X/autosome translocation in a girl with manifestations of Lowe syndrome. Am J Med Genet 23:837–847, 1986.

124. Mueller OT, Hartsfield JK, Jr., Gallardo LA, Essig Y-P, Miller KL, Papenhausen PR, et al. Lowe oculocerebrorenal syndrome in a female with a balanced X;20 translocation: mapping of the X chromosome breakpoint. Am J Hum Genet 49:804–810, 1991.

125. Xuan JY, Besner A, Ireland M, Hughes-Benzie RM, MacKenzie AE. Mapping of Simpson-Golabi-Behmel syndrome to Xq25-q27. Hum Mol Genet 3:133–137, 1994.

126. Roberts SH, Upadhyaya M, Sarfarazi M, Harper PS. Further evidence localising the gene for Hunter's syndrome to the distal region of the X chromosome long arm. J Med Genet 26:309–313, 1989.

127. Zuffardi O, Fraccaro M. Gene mapping and serendipity: the locus for torticollis, keloids, cryptorchidism and renal dysplasia (31430, McKusick) is at Xq28, distal to the G6PD locus. Hum Genet 62:280–281, 1982.

128. Hodgson SV, Neville B, Jones RWA, Fear C, Bobrow M. Two cases of X/autosome translocation in females with incontinentia pigmenti. Hum Genet 71:231–234, 1985.

129. Gilgenkrantz S, Tridon P, Pinel-Briquel N, Beurey J, Weber M. Translocation (X;9)(p11;q34) in a girl with incontinentia pigmenti (IP): implications for the regional assignment of the IP locus to Xp11? Ann Genet 28:90–92, 1985.

130. Kajii T, Tsukahara M, Fukushima Y, Hata A, Matsuo K, Kkuroki Y. Translocation (X;13)(p11.21;q12.3) in a girl with incontinentia pigmenti and bilateral retinoblastoma. Ann Genet 28:219–223, 1985.

131. Cannizzaro LA, Hecht F. Gene for incontinentia pigmenti maps to band Xp11 with an (X;10)(p11;q22) translocation. Clin Genet 32:66–69, 1987.

132. Ropers HH, Zuffardi O, Bianchi E, Tiepolo L. Agenesis of corpus callosum, ocular, and skeletal anomalies (X-linked dominant Aicardi's syndrome) in a girl with balanced X/3 translocation. Hum Genet 61:364–368, 1982.

133. Al Gazali LI, Mueller RF, Caine A, Antoniou A, McCartney A, Fitchett M, et al. Two 46,XX,t(X;Y) females with linear skin defects and congenital microphthalmia: a new syndrome at Xp22.3. J Med Genet 27:59–63, 1990.

134. Temple IK, Hurst JA, Hing S, Butler L, Baraitser M. De novo deletion of Xp22.2-

pter in a female with linear skin lesions of the face and neck, microphthalmia, and anterior chamber eye anomalies. J Med Genet 27:56–58, 1990.

135. Allanson J, Richter S. Linear skin defects and congenital microphthalmia: a new syndrome at Xp22.2. (Letter). J Med Genet 28:143–144, 1991.

136. Journel H, Melki J, Turleau C, Munnich A, de Grouchy J. Rett phenotype with X/ autosome translocation: possible mapping to the short arm of chromosome X. Am J Med Genet 35:142–147, 1990.

137. Zoghbi HY, Ledbetter DH, Schultz R, Percy AK, Glaze DG. A de novo X;3 translocation in Rett syndrome. Am J Med Genet 35:148–151, 1990.

6

Mitochondrial Inheritance

The idea that certain traits may be transmitted exclusively by the mother has existed since the 1930s. The term applied to such transmission was *cytoplasmic inheritance,* because the cytoplasm of the zygote is transmitted almost exclusively by the oocyte. The first human disease for which cytoplasmic inheritance was proposed was Leber hereditary optic neuropathy (LHON), a condition that is characterized by deterioration of the optic nerves with progressive vision loss leading to blindness. Based on the observation that almost all cases were transmitted by the mother, in 1936, Imai and Moriwaki suggested that LHON may be an example of cytoplasmic inheritance in humans.[1]

The association of cytoplasmic inheritance with mitochondrial transmission did not occur until the late 1940s when Boris Ephrussi and his co-workers conducted a series of experiments that demonstrated that the mutagenic dye euflavine produces mutations that impair the ability of the yeast cells to conduct oxidative phosphorylation.[2] Yeast bearing this mutation grow poorly, resulting in a phenotype termed *petit.* By performing cytoplasmic fusion experiments they showed that the transmission of this phenotype was through the cytoplasm rather than the nucleus. Because mitochondria mediate oxidative phosphorylation and are located in the cytoplasm, they proposed that mitochondria might contain their own genetic material. In 1950, Ephrussi and his associate Helene Hottinguer stated,

The appearance of mutant cells as a consequence of the euflavine treatment is best accounted for by assuming that an auto-reproducing cytoplasmic component, necessary for the synthesis of the respiratory enzymes in question, has not been included in some of the buds. Since a cell can alternately produce mutant and normal buds, this cytoplasmic component must be ascribed a particulate nature.[2]

Hence mitochondrial transmission was not an all-or-none phenomenon but was dependent on the genetic state of the mitochondria transferred. Proof of genetic transmission by mitochondria came in 1967 with the isolation of mitochondrial DNA (mtDNA) from human cells.[3]

The basic rules of mitochondrial transmission in humans were laid out by Robert Hersh in 1969. He stated,

There should be some properties of the mitochondria which have striking maternal inheritance. If there were a clinically manifested lesion A in the F_1 generation from a mother with A and a normal father, all progeny would have such a lesion. The F_1 daughters would transmit the disease to all progeny of the F_2 generation, but the F_1 sons would have all normal progeny provided his mate were normal.[4]

However, Hirsch overlooked the fact that an affected mother may transmit both normal and mutant mitochondria.

WHAT ARE MITOCHONDRIA?

Mitochondria are organelles in the cytoplasm of eukaryotic cells that generate cellular energy by oxidative phosphorylation.[5,6] The complexes for the electron transport chains and adenosine triphosphate (ATP) synthase are bound to the inner membrane of the mitochondria. Electrons are donated by nicotinanide-adenine dinucleotide (NADH) and by flavine-adenine dinucleotide (FADH$_2$)-containing dehydrogenases (succinate dehydrogenase, electron transfer flavo-protein dehydrogenase, and glycerol-3-phosphate dehydrogenase) to the four complexes that make up the electron transport chain. As the electrons are transported by complexes I, III, and IV, protons are pumped across the mitochondrial inner membrane. This creates an electrochemical gradient that is used by ATP synthase to combine adenosine diphosphate and inorganic phosphate (ADP and Pi). Intermediate steps in other metabolic pathways, including the Krebs tricarboxylic acid and the urea cycles and the oxidation of medium chain fatty acids, are carried out in mitochondria.

STRUCTURE OF THE HUMAN MITOCHONDRIAL GENOME

The human mitochondrial genome has several properties that differ from those of the nuclear genome.[6] These include cytoplasmic compartmentalization, a compact structure, and a unique genetic code. The mitochondrial genome contains the information for seven subunits of NADH dehydrogenase (complex I), the apocytochrome b component of ubinquinol cytochrome c reductase (complex III), three subunits of cytochrome c oxidase (complex IV), and two subunits of ATP synthase (complex V). In addition the mitochondrial genome encodes the genes for 12s and 16s ribosomal subunits and 22 transfer RNAs (tRNAs) for translation of the mitochondrial genome products. The genes encoding the tRNAs are located between the genes encoding the mitochondrial proteins (Fig. 6.1).

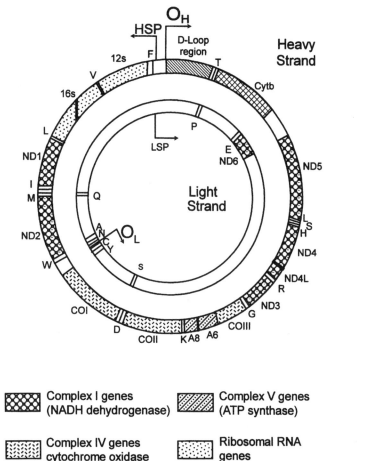

Figure 6.1. Structure of the mitochondrial genome. The origins of replication for the light and heavy strands are indicated by O_L and O_H, respectively. LSP indicates light-strand promoter and HSP indicates heavy-strand promoter. The transfer RNA genes are indicated by single letters. Genes corresponding to the various complexes are indicated by the different forms of shading.[7]

DNA sequence. The complete sequence of human mt DNA was determined by Barrell and his co-workers in 1981.[7] The human mitochondrial genome is a double-stranded DNA molecule that is 16,569 base pairs in length. Most of the molecule is comprised of coding sequences. The DNA molecule has a purine-rich adenine and guanine (A&G) heavy strand and a pyrimidine-rich cytidine and thymidine (C&T) light strand, each with its own origin of replication. The replication of the two strands is asynchronous, resulting in a triple-stranded region known as a displacement (or D) loop.[8,9] This region is displaced by the synthesis of a short piece of heavy strand (7s) DNA.[8,9] The human mitochondrial genome is more compact and mitochondrial genes have no intervening sequences (Fig. 6.1).[9]

Structure of mitochondria in other species. The structure of mitochondrial DNA from many organisms has been characterized. The size of the mitochondrial genomes in other animal species is comparable to that in humans.[10] In yeast the size of the mitochondrial genome may be up to five times greater and in plants up to 20 times greater than in humans.[11] The rate of mutation in the human mitochondrial genome is at least ten times higher than that in the nuclear genome.[12,13] This may reflect a higher rate of oxidative damage from superoxide exposure, an error-prone DNA replication system, an absence of repair systems comparable to those in the nucleus, or the lack of a recombinational mechanism. The presence of the mitochondrial form of superoxide dismutase may favor the development of free radicals and promote mutation. A high proportion of silent to replacement substitutions suggests that selection occurs against functional changes at the protein level. Short tandemly repeated sequences may predispose to some of the deletional mutational events that occur in the mitochondrial genome.[14–18]

Genetic code. In mammals, the mitochondrial genome has a unique genetic code that varies from that in the nucleus.[7,19] Codon differences include ATA for methionine (instead of ATG), TGA for tryptophan (instead of TGG), and AGA and AGG for stop (instead of TAG, TGA, and TGT). This genetic code resembles that in archaebacteria, specifically α-purple bacteria.[20] The structure of the mitochondria and the mitochondrial genetic code suggest that these organelles had an independent origin as free-living organisms.[21,22] Subsequently they were engulfed by early eukaryotic cells, providing these cells with the machinery for aerobic metabolism. Mitochondria thus survive as endosymbionts, providing some essential functions to the host and having most of their proteins encoded by nuclear genes and transported from the cytoplasm across the mitochondrial membranes. It is unknown whether mitochondria have had a single or multiple independent evolutionary origins.[20]

Transfer of genes to the nuclear genome. During the course of evolution, genes were transferred to the nucleus and potentially lost from the mitochondrial genome. In humans DNA sequences complementary to the mitochondrial genome have been found in the nuclear genome. These include part of the 12S ribosomal RNA gene, the cytochrome c oxidase I gene and two NADH dehydrogenase genes. These sequences have not been found in the nuclear genomes of other primates, suggesting a recent origin.[23]

Mitochondrial polymorphisms. Naturally occurring mitochondrial DNA polymorphisms have been identified.[12,13,24] These polymorphisms correlate with the ethnic and geographic origin of the subjects who have been studied. They have been used to develop phylogenetic trees for human populations. Based on such observations, Wilson and co-workers proposed that humans descended from a common evolutionary ancestor,[25] a hypothesis that has been disputed by others.[26]

MITOCHONDRIAL GENETICS

Every cell contains hundreds of mitochondria. Each mitochondrion contains four to five genomes.[27,28] Mitochondria are transmitted from mothers to their progeny through the oocytes, which contain thousands of these organelles. Spermatocytes have far fewer mitochondria than oocytes. The contribution of mitochondria by spermatocytes is estimated to be less than 1% of the total in the zygote.[29] Matrilineal inheritance of mitochondrial DNA (mtDNA) was demonstrated by the maternal transmission of polymorphic mtDNA restriction fragment patterns.[24,30] This pattern of inheritance is different from X-linked inheritance because there is no father-to-daughter transmission (Fig. 6.2). Experimentally, mitochondrial transmission can be demonstrated by cytoplasmic transmission of a trait. Such transmission has been demonstrated for chloramphenicol resistance.[31–33]

Heteroplasmy. Mitochondria may be mosaic for mutations that affect some, but not all, copies of the mitochondrial genome; thus, a subset of mitochondrial genomes within a cell may carry a mutation, a condition that is known as *heteroplasmy* (Fig. 6.3).[29,34] Heteroplasmy for mitochondrial mutations may vary among siblings and even among tissues in an individual. The factors that

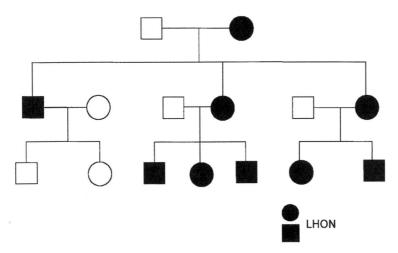

Figure 6.2. Pedigree with Leber hereditary optic neuropathy demonstrating maternal transmission.

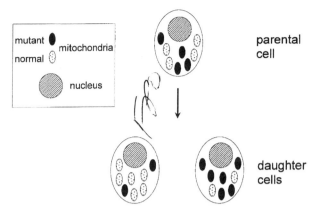

Figure 6.3. Demonstration of heteroplasmy in mitochondria. As the result of unequal partitioning of mitochondrial genomes, the genetic constitution of can vary between the mitochondria of the parental and the daughter cells.

affect this are unequal partitioning of mitochondria during meiosis and mitosis and possible selective replication of shortened (deleted) mitochondrial genomes. Requirements for compatibility with the host cell may also affect the viability of mitochondrial genomes in unknown ways.[35] For example, proteins that are encoded in the mitochondrial genome must be able to assemble and function with proteins that are encoded in the host genome.

Correlation with phenotype. Mutations in the mitochondrial genome occur as the result of point mutations, as well as deletions and duplications.[36] These mutations are likely to affect oxidative phosphorylation. The tissues that sustain damage from mutations in the mitochondrial genome are those for which oxidative phosphorylation is the main source of energy, including brain, muscle, heart, liver, kidney, and islet cells of the pancreas. These tissues are the most susceptible to ischemia from hypoperfusion and from uncoupling of oxidative phosphorylation by such agents as cyanide, dinitrophenol, and azide. Ischemia in muscle produces a mitochondrial myopathy characterized histologically by ragged red fibers, that is, degenerating type I fibers that accumulate aggregates of abnormal mitochondria. Both the tissue distribution and the degree of heteroplasmy within a given tissue may affect the phenotype. Criteria for associating a point mutation with a particular phenotype include (1) presence in a high proportion of mitochondria in a given individual, (2) alteration of a codon that is highly conserved among species, and (3) presence in a high proportion of individuals with that phenotype and few unaffected maternal relatives of the affected family members.

Point mutations. Point mutations in mitochondria are characterized by a high proportion of silent versus replacement substitutions (>90% versus <10%), a high transition to transversion ratio (10:1), and a strong bias toward C/T transitions in the L strand.[20] New mutations may occur as the result of oxidative damage to the mitochondrial DNA. Hotspots for point mutations, such as the CG dinucleotides in the nuclear genome, have not been observed in the mitochondrial genome. Point mutations in the mitochondrial genome are often inherited. Matrilinear family members that inherit the same point mutation may demonstrate similar phenotypes.

Point mutation in the coding regions. Leber hereditary optic neuropathy (LHON) is associated not only with progressive vision loss and blindness but also with cardiac arrhythmia.[37–41] The peak age of onset of disease is during the second and third decades of life. The first LHON mutation was identified by Douglas Wallace.[42] This mutation, the substitution of a guanine for an adenine at position 11,778, results in the replacement of an arginine for a histidine at codon 340 of the ND4 subunit of complex I. (This histidine residue is conserved in all species for which the ND4 subunit gene has been sequenced.)[42] The mutation has been found in about 50% of individuals with LHON and in no unaffected control individuals. The mutation has occurred on several different genetic backgrounds (*haplotypes*) suggesting multiple origins.[43] In some large pedigrees the mutation is homoplasmic in multiple generations. In other pedigrees and in singleton cases, the mutation-bearing mitochondrial genome is heteroplasmic, with the degree of heteroplasmy varying among individuals and among tissues in affected individuals.[44,45]

Other mutations in the mitochondrial genome have been associated with LHON because they are found in a much higher proportion of affected individuals than unaffected controls, and they alter an evolutionarily conserved amino acid residue.[46–54] These have been found in the genes that encode electron transport subunit complexes I, III, and IV. Some mutations are sufficient to produce disease. Others operate in association with each other or with the 11,778 mutation to affect the penetrance of the disease (Table 6.1). In one large pedigree, four mutations were found to accumulate sequentially. With the occurrence of each new mutation, the likelihood of blindness increased (Table 6.1).[36,50]

The genetics of Leber hereditary optic atrophy are unusual. Among Europeans, 84% of affected individuals are male, whereas among Japanese, 59% are male.[55] The age of onset is lower and the penetrance is higher among male offspring than among female offspring who receive the mutation from their mothers. Factors that may influence expression of the disease phenotype are the different mutations and their interactions, the degree of heteroplasmy in the susceptible tissue, and possible interactions with mitochondrial proteins that are encoded in the nucleus. The fact that mutations in different subunits of different complexes can result in the LHON phenotype and that mutations may be cumulative suggests that the disorder is caused by impairment of oxidative phosphorylation rather than loss of a particular enzyme or subunit.

Because nuclear genes encode most of the subunits involved in oxidative phosphorylation, some have suggested that nuclear genes, especially on the X chromosome, may account for the sex-related differences in the penetrance of

Table 6.1. Mutations in Leber Hereditary Optic Atrophy

Locus	Position	Nucleotide	Amino acid
Sufficient to produce disease			
ND1	3,460	G→A	A→T
ND1	4,160	T→C	L→P
CYB1	5,257	G→A	D→N
Interact to increase penetrance			
ND1	4,216	T→C	Y→H
ND2	4,917	A→G	D→N
ND2	5,244	G→A	G→S
ND5	13,708	G→A	A→T
CYB	15,812	G→A	V→M
Sequential mutations increasing penetrance			
ND5	13,708	G→A	A→T
CYB	15,257	G→A	D→N
CYB	15,812	G→A	V→M
ND2	5,244	G→A	G→S

LHON.[56] Such a two locus model (one mitochondrial, one X chromosomal) fit the observed penetrance of LHON in three affected families.[57] Linkage disequilibrium with markers at DXS7 suggests a possible site for this nuclear-encoded locus.[58] Alternatively, the development of LHON could be a sex-limited trait, with males having a higher metabolic rate in the optic nerve, or males may have different environmental exposures, for example, carbon monoxide in cigarette smoke. The optic nerve degeneration in LHON is a progressive process that may result from the additive effects of genetic and environmental insults to oxidative phosphorylation.

Point mutations in the mitochondrial genome have been associated with other diseases. A missense mutation at nucleotide 8993 (T→G, resulting in substitution of arginine for leucine) has been associated with neurogenic muscle weakness, ataxia, and retinitis pigmentosa (NARP),[59] and with Leigh disease, a lethal childhood condition with degeneration of the basal ganglia.[60] NARP showed maternal transmission and the severity correlated with the fraction of mutant RNA molecules.

Point mutations in tRNA genes. Mutations in the transfer RNA (tRNA) genes decrease mitochondrial protein synthesis.[61] These mutations usually have more systemic manifestations than point mutations in specific subunits. The activities of complexes I and IV, that is, those with the greatest number of mitochondrially encoded subunits, are the most affected. The susceptible tissues include skeletal muscle, heart, and nerve. The severity of the clinical disorder may correlate with the degree of the oxidative phosphorylation defect.[62] The resulting impairment of glycolysis may be so severe that lactic acidosis may serve as a marker for mitochondrial disease.

Mitochondrial myopathy, encephalopathy, lactic acidosis, and stroke-like episodes (MELAS) are associated with episodic vomiting, seizures, and recurrent but reversible cerebral insults producing cortical blindness, hemiparesis, and hemianopsia.[63-65] A mutation at position 3243 in the dihydrouridine loop of the mitochondrial tRNA-leu gene has been found in 80% of cases of MELAS.[66-68] In vitro, this mutation also inactivates the transcription terminator for the rRNA genes; thus, both the ratio of mRNA and rRNA transcripts and the efficiency of translation may be altered.[69,70] Maternal relatives may have only subtle neurologic abnormalities, although these may worsen with age. The proportion of mutant genomes is higher in the cells of severely affected individuals than in the cells of their unaffected or their mildly affected relatives. The ragged red fibers in this condition occur in cells in which there is a high proportion of mutant mitochondrial genomes.[63-65,71,72]

Myoclonic epilepsy with ragged red fibers (MERFF) demonstrates maternal transmission. Expression among maternal relatives is variable; the most severely affected have dementia, neurosensory hearing loss, myoclonus, cardiomyopathy, and renal dysfunction. Individuals start off normal in life and worsen with age.[62,73] A mutation is the tRNA-lys gene at position 8344 in the $T\psi C$ loop has been found in three independent pedigrees.[62,74-77] This reduces mitochondrial protein synthesis and preferentially affects the activities of complexes I and IV. The age of onset correlates with the proportion of mutant mitochondrial genomes in affected individuals. Treatment with coenzyme Q has been shown to result in clinical improvement of some affected individuals.[62,78]

Two other disorders have been associated with mutations in mitochondrial tRNA genes. Maternally inherited myopathy and cardiomyopathy is associated with a mutation in the tRNA-leu (UUR) gene at position 3260 in the stem of the anticodon loop. This mutation is associated with defects in complexes I and IV of the electron transport chain.[79] Lethal infantile cardiomyopathy is associated with failure to thrive, hypotonia, and death from cardiomyopathy within a few months of birth. In one case, a mutation was observed at position 4317 in the tRNA-Ile gene and in two other cases at positions 15,923 and 15,924 in the anticodon loops of the tRNA-Thr gene.[80,81]

Point mutations in rRNA genes. The susceptibility of mammalian cells to the toxic effects of the antibiotic chloramphenicol is mediated by the mitochondrial genome.[31-33] Chloramphenicol exerts its antibiotic effect in bacteria by attaching to the large ribosomal subunit, thereby preventing this subunit from binding to the smaller subunit. In keeping with their bacterial origin, chloramphenicol has a similar effect in mitochondria. Eukaryotic cell lines have been identified that are resistant to the effects of chloramphenicol, both natural variants and those that were created by using ethidium bromide as a mutagen. This resistance was transmitted experimentally to susceptible cells by fusing enucleated cybrids. The resistance in human, mouse, and yeast mitochondria resulted from mutations in the chloramphenicol binding site of the 16s (large subunit) ribosomal subunit.[82,83]

In humans, two types of chloramphenicol toxicity have been observed, dose-related and idiosyncratic. Dose-related toxicity can be demonstrated in all individuals. Idiosyncratic toxicity occurs in approximately one in 19,000 individuals. The susceptibility phenotype is maternally transmitted. In one case, identical twins were affected, and in another a man and his sister's daughter.[84,85] To date, specific mutations have not been identified that confer idiosyncratic sensitivity. In individuals who recover from chloramphenicol toxicity, selection for chloramphenicol resistance takes place in the bone marrow cells as judged by their viability to in vitro exposure to the antibiotic.[86]

Exposure to aminoglycosides, streptomycin, gentamicin, kanamycin, and tobramycin causes ototoxicity and deafness in some susceptible individuals. The mechanism of toxicity is thought to be interference with the production of ATP in the mitochondria of the hair cells of the cochlea. In most pedigrees with multiple affected individuals in several generations, the susceptibility to antibiotic toxicity is transmitted by the females exclusively. Although this finding is consistent with mitochondrial transmission, to date a specific mutation has not been identified in the mitochondrial genome.[87,88]

Deletions and duplications. Most mitochondrial deletions occur as new events in germ or somatic cells. This means that family members frequently do not manifest the phenotype of the affected individual.[89] Deletions can occur throughout a person's lifetime.[90] The deletions are propagated in the cell lines in which they arose.[91] The time at which the mutation occurred affects the distribution of the mutation in the tissues. Germline mutations affect multiple tissues, whereas somatic mutations may affect a limited number of tissues. The phenotype can vary, depending on the cell lines that carry the deletion and the degree of heteroplasmy in those tissues.[90–97]

Over 100 deletions have been described that remove tRNA, rRNA, and structural subunit coding genes. Most spare the origins of replication of the heavy and light strands and the light-strand promoter. Some deletions remove the heavy-strand promoter, suggesting that is not necessary for maintenance of mitochondrial DNA.[36] The most common deletions occur between direct repeats in the mitochondrial genome. One hotspot is at nucleotides 8468 and 13,446. Slip replication is the favored model for at least some deletions. This occurs if the upstream repeat on the displaced H strand pairs with the downstream repeat on the L strand when it is exposed by the replication fork. If the single stranded loop from the H strand then breaks, the sequences between the two direct repeats are then lost (Fig. 6.4).[18,90] Nuclear genes that encode the mitochondrial DNA replication enzymes may affect the occurrence of mitochondrial deletions.[98]

There may be several molecular consequences of the deletions. The deletions involve a number of tRNA genes. This may have the effect of decreasing the translation of all subunits of the respiratory chain that are encoded in mitochondria. In addition, although the mRNAs from the deleted mtDNA molecule may be transcribed, this RNA is either not translated or is rapidly degraded.[92,99]

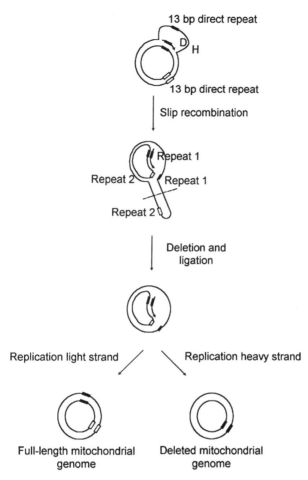

13 bp direct repeat

13 bp direct repeat

Slip recombination

Repeat 1

Repeat 2   Repeat 1

Repeat 2

Deletion and
ligation

Replication light strand   Replication heavy strand

Full-length mitochondrial   Deleted mitochondrial
genome   genome

Figure 6.4. Mechanism of deletion of mitochondrial genomes by slip recombination during replication.

Two tissues that are most susceptible to aerobic damage from germline mitochondrial deletions are the retina and skeletal muscle, especially the external ocular muscles. Damage to this muscle group results in weakness of eye movements or chronic progressive external ophthalmoplegia. In many instances this damage may occur over a span of years before the clinical features of the disease are manifested.[100] The clinical or biochemical severity does not correlate with the proportion of deleted mtDNAs in the muscle studied.[95,101]

Two conditions that have been associated with mitochondrial deletions are Kearn-Sayre syndrome (more recently termed *ocular myopathy*) and Pearson bone marrow–pancreas syndrome.[102,103] Kearn-Sayre syndrome is a condition of chronic progressive external ophthalmoplegia with cardiomyopathy and pigmentary degeneration of the retina. The Pearson bone marrow–pancreas syn-

drome is characterized by refractory sideroblastic anemia and exocrine pancreatic dysfunction. Severe transfusion dependent macrocytic anemia develops
during infancy, as does pancreatic fibrosis. Patients who survive Pearson syndrome have gone on to develop features of Kearn-Sayre syndrome and Leigh
disease.[104,105]

Duplications of the mitochondrial genome have been found in two sporadic
cases of mitochondrial myopathy and in one familial case.[106–108] These cases
were associated with diabetes mellitus, ptosis, chronic progressive external ophthalmoplegia, retinopathy, ataxia, deafness, and proximal renal tubular acidosis.
In the sporadic cases the sizes of the duplicated segments were 7.6 and 8.0 kb,
respectively, and interrupted a duplicated segment of the gene for the first subunit of cytochrome oxidase. In the familial case, the duplicated segment was
10 kb in length and joined duplicated regions of the cytochrome *b* and ATPase
genes. The mechanism of duplication may have involved circular dimerization
during replication with subsequent deletion by recombination between homologous segments or breakage and joining between nonhomologous segments. The
identification of 3- and 4-bp direct repeats, respectively, at the boundaries of
the deleted regions for the sporadic and familial cases is compatible with recombination between homologous segments.

MITOCHONDRIAL DISORDERS WITH AUTOSOMAL
DOMINANT TRANSMISSION

An exception to maternal transmission of disorders affecting mitochondria has
been found in several pedigrees.[98,109–111] These individuals had chronic progressive external ophthalmoplegia, proximal muscle wasting, and sensorineural
hearing loss. The symptoms progressed steadily with aging. Muscle biopsies
showed ragged red fibers, and complex I and IV activities were reduced to 50%
of normal. Based on transmission from both mother and father to offspring,
these pedigrees showed autosomal dominant inheritance. Affected individuals
had multiple different mtDNA deletions. All of the deletions were flanked by
direct repeats although the repeats were frequently imperfect and frequently
were very short (three or four bases). Massimo Zeviani has suggested that the
mechanism by which multiple mtDNA deletions are produced may be identical
or similar to that by which single mutations are induced (e.g., slip replication)
but that the frequency of events is increased. Alternatively, the genetic abnormality could be in a hypothetical factor devoted to selecting and eliminating
abnormal mtDNAs. Based on the pattern of inheritance, the mutations are likely
to be nuclear-encoded genes.[111]

LATE SOMATIC MITOCHONDRIAL MUTATION

There is a decline in respiratory function in skeletal muscle with increasing
age.[112] Wallace has suggested that each individual is born with an initial capac-

ity for oxidative phosphorylation. When this capacity falls below the threshold of requirement of ATP generation for a given organ, disease symptoms appear.[113] Individuals who are born with mutations in their mitochondrial genomes start off with a lower threshold for oxidative phosphorylation than others. One way that this threshold is lowered is through the progressive accumulation of mitochondrial mutations over life. In this way, mitochondrial mutation becomes part of the normal aging process, although it may be accelerated as the result of other mutations in the mitochondrial or nuclear genomes or from the exposure to environmental mutagens. In two studies, the percentage of hearts with 7.4-kb deletions increased with age.[114,115] In another study, the quantity of mitochondrial genomes with 5-kb deletions in histologically normal hearts increased with age.[116] The 5-kb deletion has not been detected in the brains of normal children but has been found in the brains of adults.[116] The deletion analyses assay a small proportion of mutations in mitochondrial genomes. The degree of mutation in the mitochondrial genomes of in the tissues of elderly adults may prove to be quite large.

Coronary artery disease is associated with ischemia of the heart muscle. This has been associated with an increased frequency of deletion and with induction of transcription of both nuclear and mitochondrial genes.[117–119] Coronary artery disease may act as a vicious cycle with ischemia promoting mitochondrial mutation and worsening the ischemia and potentially the heart failure.[120] Because mitochondria continue to replicate even in nondividing cells, the accumulation of deleterious mutations may limit the lifespan of humans.[121]

Some neurodegenerative diseases are late-onset, generally sporadic in occurrence, and associated with defects in oxidative phosphorylation. Parkinson disease is a late-onset movement disorder that is associated with loss of dopaminergic neurons in the substantia nigra. Oxidative phosphorylation defects have been demonstrated in the brain, muscle, and platelets of affected individuals. These are heterogeneous in nature.[122–126] In one study of six patients, two had complex I defects, one had a complex IV defect, two had complex I and complex III defects. The other two had normal activity.[127,128] Deletions and point mutations of mitochondrial DNA have been identified in the brains of Parkinson disease patients, although the significance of these mutations has been disputed because they may simply represent age-related effects.[129–132] An experimental model of Parkinson disease can be induced by treatment with the inhibitor of oxidative phosphorylation, 1-methyl1-4-phenyl-1,2,3,6-tetrahydropyridine (MPTP).[133] This provides further evidence for mitochondrial dysfunction in some, if not all, patients.

Alzheimer disease is generally sporadic in occurrence, although familial cases with autosomal dominant transmission have been described. Mutations in the genes for complex I and IV have been found in the brains of individuals with Alzheimer disease; thus, it has been suggested that some forms of Alzheimer disease may be mediated by mitochondria.[134,135]

Mitochondria are maternally transmitted and contain their own genetic information. Mutations in the mitochondrial genome can be either inherited or acquired. Inherited mutations are associated with maternal transmission of the disease phenotype. The likelihood that a given mutation will produce disease is determined by the gene that it disrupts, the function of mitochondrial genomes in a given cell that contains the mutation, and the specific cell types that are affected. Because mutations accumulate with aging, mitochondrial dysfunction is a feature of several adult-onset conditions, including coronary artery and neurodegenerative diseases. Hence, mitochondria act as genetic modifiers.

Even with the identification of mitochondrial transmission, not all of the cases of preferential parental transmission had been identified. Some traits are not Y-linked, but show preferential paternal transmission. Some traits that are not X-linked or encoded on the mitochondrial genome show preferential maternal transmission. The general term that was developed for this concept is *genomic imprinting*.

REFERENCES

1. Imai Y, Moriwaki D. A probable case of cytoplasmic inheritance in man: a critique of Leber's disease. J Genet Hum 33:136–167, 1936.
2. Ephrussi B, Hotinguer H. Direct demonstration of the mutagenic action of euflavine on baker's yeast. Nature 166:956–958, 1950.
3. Clayton DA, Vinograd J. Circular dimer and catenate forms of mitochondrial DNA in human leukaemic leukocytes. Nature 216:652–657, 1967.
4. Hersh RT. Mitochondrial genetics: a conjecture. Science 166:402, 1969.
5. Attardi G, Schatz G. Biogenesis of mitochondria. Annu. Rev Cell Biol 4:289–333, 1988.
6. Tzagoloff A, Myers AM. Genetics of mitochondrial biogenesis. Annu Rev Biochem 55:249–285, 1992.
7. Anderson S, Bankier AT, Barrell BG, de Bruijn MHL, Coulson AR, Drouin J, et al. Sequence and organization of the human mitochondrial genome. Nature 290:457–465, 1981.
8. Clayton DA. Replication of animal mitochondrial DNA. Cell 28:693–705, 1982.
9. Clayton DA. Transcription of the mitochondrial genome. Annu Rev Biochem 53:573–594, 1984.
10. Attardi G. Animal mitochondrial DNA: an extreme example of genetic economy. Int Rev Cytol 93:93–145, 1985.
11. Wolf K, Del Giudice L. The variable mitochondrial genome of ascomycetes: organization, mutational alterations, and expression. Adv Genet 25:185–308, 1992.
12. Cann RL, Wilson AC. Length mutations in human mitochondrial DNA. Genetics 104:699–711, 1983.
13. Cann RL, Brown WM, Wilson AC. Polymorphic sites and the mechanism of evolution in human mitochondrial DNA. Genetics 106:479–499, 1984.
14. Mita S, Rizzuto R, Moraes CT, Shanske S, Arnaudo E, Fabrizi GM, et al. Recombination via flanking direct repeats is a major cause of large-scale deletions of human mitochondrial DNA. Nucleic Acids Res 18:561–567, 1990.
15. Johns DR, Rutledge SL, Stine OC, Hurko O. Directly repeated sequences associated with pathogenic mitochondrial DNA deletions. Proc Natl Acad Sci USA 86:8059–8062, 1989.
16. Nelson I, Degoul F, Obermaier Kusser B, Romero N, Borrone C, Marsac C, et al.

Mapping of heteroplasmic mitochondrial DNA deletions in Kearns-Sayre syndrome. Nucleic Acids Res 17:8117–8124, 1989.

17. Holt IJ, Harding AE, Morgan Hughes JA. Deletions of muscle mitochondrial DNA in mitochondrial myopathies: sequence analysis and possible mechanisms. Nucleic Acids Res 17:4465–4469, 1989.

18. Schon EA, Rizzuto R, Moraes CT, Nakase H, Zeviani M, Dimauro S. A direct repeat is a hotspot for large-scale deletion of human mitochondrial DNA. Science 244:346–349, 1989.

19. Barrell BG, Bankier AT, Drouin J. A different genetic code in human mitochondria. Nature 282:189–194, 1979.

20. Gray MW. Origin and evolution of mitochondrial DNA. Annu Rev Cell Biol 5:25–50, 1989.

21. Gray MW, Sankoff D, Cedergren RJ. On the evolutionary descent of organisms and organelles: a global phylogeny based on a highly conserved structural core in small subunit ribosomal RNA. Nucleic Acids Res 12:5837–5852, 1984.

22. Spencer DF, Schnare MN, Gray MW. Pronounced structural similarity between the small subunit ribosomal RNA genes of wheat mitochondria and Escherichia coli. Proc Natl Acad Sci USA 81:493–497, 1984.

23. Kamimura N, Ishii S, Ma LD, Shay JW. Three separate mitochondrial DNA sequences are contiguous in human genomic DNA. J Mol Biol 210:703–707, 1989.

24. Case JT, Wallace DC. Maternal inheritance of mitochondrial DNA polymorphisms in cultured human fibroblasts. Somat Cell Genet 7:103–108, 1981.

25. Cann RL, Stoneking M, Wilson AC. Mitochondrial DNA and human evolution. Nature 325:31–36, 1987.

26. Kruger J, Vogel F. The problem of our common mitochondrial mother. Hum Genet 82:308–312, 1989.

27. Bogenhagen D, Clayton DA. The number of mitochondrial deoxyribonucleic acid genomes in mouse L and human HeLa cells. J Biol Chem 249:7991–7995, 1974.

28. Oliver NA, Wallace DC. Assignment of two mitochondrially synthesized polypeptides to human mitochondrial DNA and their use in the study of intracellular mitochondrial interaction. Mol Cell Biol 2:30–41, 1982.

29. Michaels GS, Hauswirth WW, Laipis PJ. Mitochondrial DNA copy number in bovine oocytes and somatic cells. Dev Biol 94:246–251, 1982.

30. Giles RE, Blanc H, Cann HM, Wallace DC. Maternal inheritance of human mitochondrial DNA. Proc Natl Acad Sci USA 77:6715–6719, 1980.

31. Bunn CL, Wallace DC, Eisenstadt JM. Cytoplasmic inheritance of chloramphenicol resistance in mouse tissue culture cells. Proc Natl Acad Sci USA 71:1681–1684, 1974.

32. Wallace DC, Bunn CL, Eisenstadt JM. Cytoplasmic transfer of chloramphenicol resistance in human tissue culture cells. J Cell Biol 67:174–188, 1975.

33. Wallace DC. Mitotic segregation of mitochondrial DNAs in human cell hybrids and expression of chloramphenicol resistance. Somat Cell Mol Genet 12:41–49, 1986.

34. Howell N, Huang P, Kolodner RD. Origin, transmission, and segregation of mitochondrial DNA dimers in mouse hybrid and cybrid cell lines. Somat Cell Mol Genet 10:259–274, 1984.

35. Shay JW, Ishii S. Unexpected nonrandom mitochondrial DNA segregation in human cell hybrids. Anticancer Res 10:279–284, 1990.

36. Wallace DC. Diseases of the mitochondrial DNA. Annu Rev Biochem 61:1175–1212, 1992.

37. Wilson J. Leber's hereditary optic atrophy: some clinical and aetiological considerations. Brain 86:347–362, 1963.

38. Nikoskelainen E. New aspects of the genetic, etiologic, and clinical puzzle of Leber's disease. Neurology 34:1482–1484, 1984.

39. Newman NJ, Wallace DC. Mitochondria and Leber's hereditary optic neuropathy. Am J Ophthalmol 109:726–730, 1990.

40. Nikoskelainen E, Wanne O, Dahl M. Pre-excitation syndrome and Leber's hereditary optic neuroretinopathy. Lancet 1:696, 1985.

41. Bower SP, Hawley I, Mackey DA. Cardiac arrhythmia and Leber's hereditary optic neuropathy. Lancet 339:1427–1428, 1992.

42. Wallace DC, Singh G, Lott MT, Hodge JA, Schurr TG, Lezza AM, et al. Mitochondrial DNA mutation associated with Leber's hereditary optic neuropathy. Science 242:1427–1430, 1988.

43. Singh G, Lott MT, Wallace DC. A mitochondrial DNA mutation as a cause of Leber's hereditary optic neuropathy. N Engl J Med 320:1300–1305, 1989.

44. Lott MT, Voljavec AS, Wallace DC. Variable genotype of Leber's hereditary optic neuropathy patients. Am J Ophthalmol 109:625–631, 1990.

45. Holt IJ, Miller DH, Harding AE. Genetic heterogeneity and mitochondrial DNA heteroplasmy in Leber's hereditary optic neuropathy. J Med Genet 26:739–743, 1989.

46. Howell N, Bindoff LA, McCullough DA, Kubacka I, Poulton J, Mackey D, et al. Leber hereditary optic neuropathy: identification of the same mitochondrial ND1 mutation in six pedigrees. Am J Hum Genet 49:939–950, 1991.

47. Huoponen K, Vilkki J, Aula P, Nikoskelainen EK, Savontaus ML. A new mtDNA mutation associated with Leber hereditary optic neuroretinopathy. Am J Hum Genet 48:1147–1153, 1991.

48. Howell N, Kubacka I, Xu M, McCullough DA. Leber hereditary optic neuropathy: involvement of the mitochondrial ND1 gene and evidence for an intragenic suppressor mutation. Am J Hum Genet 48:935–942, 1991.

49. Johns DR, Berman J. Alternative, simultaneous complex I mitochondrial DNA mutations in Leber's hereditary optic neuropathy. Biochem Biophys Res Commun 174:1324–1330, 1991.

50. Brown MD, Voljavec AS, Lott MT, Torroni A, Yang CC, Wallace DC. Mitochondrial DNA complex I and III mutations associated with Leber's hereditary optic neuropathy. Genetics 130:163–173, 1992.

51. Majander A, Huoponen K, Savontaus ML, Nikoskelainen E, Wikstrom M. Electron transfer properties of NADH:ubiquinone reductase in the ND1/3460 and the ND4/11778 mutations of the Leber hereditary optic neuroretinopathy (LHON). FEBS Lett 292:289–292, 1991.

52. Johns DR, Neufeld MJ. Cytochrome b mutations in Leber hereditary optic neuropathy. Biochem Biophys Res Commun 181:1358–1364, 1991.

53. Johns DR. Mitochondrial ND-I mutation in Leber hereditary optic neuropathy. Am J Hum Genet 50:872–874, 1992.

54. Brown MD, Yang CC, Trounce I, Torroni A, Lott MT, Wallace DC. A mitochondrial DNA variant, identified in Leber hereditary optic neuropathy patients, which extends the amino acid sequence of cytochrome c oxidase subunit I. Am J Hum Genet 51:378–385, 1992.

55. McKusick VA. Mendelian Inheritance in Man. 8th ed. Baltimore: Johns Hopkins University Press, 1988.

56. Chen JD, Denton MJ. X-chromosomal gene in Leber hereditary optic neuroretinopathy. Am J Hum Genet 49:692–693, 1991.

57. Bu XD, Rotter JI. X chromosome-linked and mitochondrial gene control of Leber hereditary optic neuropathy: evidence from segregation analysis for dependence on X chromosome inactivation. Proc Natl Acad Sci USA 88:8198–8202, 1991.

58. Vilkki J, Ott J, Savontaus ML, Aula P, Nikoskelainen EK. Optic atrophy in Leber hereditary optic neuroretinopathy is probably determined by an X-chromosomal gene closely linked to DXS7. Am J Hum Genet 48:486–491, 1991.

59. Holt IJ, Harding AE, Petty RK, Morgan Hughes JA. A new mitochondrial disease associated with mitochondrial DNA heteroplasmy. Am J Hum Genet 46:428–433, 1990.

60. Tatuch Y, Christodoulou J, Feigenbaum A, Clarke JT, Wherret J, Smith C, et al. Heteroplasmic mtDNA mutation (T-G) at 8993 can cause Leigh disease when the percentage of abnormal mtDNA is high. Am J Hum Genet 50:852–858, 1992.

61. Wallace DC, Lott MT, Shoffner JM, Brown MD. Diseases resulting from mitochondrial DNA point mutations. J Inherit Metab Dis 15:472–479, 1992.

62. Wallace DC, Zheng XX, Lott MT, Shoffner JM, Hodge JA, Kelley RI, et al. Familial mitochondrial encephalomyopathy (MERRF): genetic, pathophysiological, and biochemical characterization of a mitochondrial DNA disease. Cell 55:601–610, 1988.

63. Moraes CT, Ricci E, Bonilla E, Dimauro S, Schon EA. The mitochondrial tRNA (Leu(UUR)) mutation in mitochondrial encephalomyopathy, lactic acidosis, and strokelike episodes (MELAS): genetic, biochemical, and morphological correlations in skeletal muscle. Am J Hum Genet 50:934–949, 1992.

64. Ciafaloni E, Ricci E, Shanske S, Moraes CT, Silvestri G, Hirano M, et al. MELAS: clinical features, biochemistry, and molecular genetics. Ann Neurol 31:391–398, 1992.

65. Goto Y, Horai S, Matsuoka T, Koga Y, Nihei K, Kobayashi M, et al. Mitochondrial myopathy, encephalopathy, lactic acidosis, and stroke-like episodes (MELAS): a correlative study of the clinical features and mitochondrial DNA mutation. Neurology 42:545–550, 1992.

66. Goto Y, Nonaka I, Horai S. A mutation in the tRNA(Leu)(UUR) gene associated with the MELAS subgroup of mitochondrial encephalomyopathies. Nature 348:651–653, 1990.

67. Kobayashi Y, Momoi MY, Tominaga K, Shimoizumi H, Nihei K, Yanagisawa M, et al. Respiration-deficient cells are caused by a single point mutation in the mitochondrial tRNA-Leu (UUR) gene in mitochondrial myopathy, encephalopathy, lactic acidosis, and strokelike episodes (MELAS). Am J Hum Genet 49:590–599, 1991.

68. Enter C, Muller Hocker J, Zierz S, Kurlemann G, Pongratz D, Forster C, et al. A specific point mutation in the mitochondrial genome of Caucasians with MELAS. Hum Genet 88:233–236, 1991.

69. Hess JF, Parisi MA, Bennett JL, Clayton DA. Impairment of mitochondrial transcription termination by a point mutation associated with the MELAS subgroup of mitochondrial encephalomyopathies. Nature 351:236–239, 1991.

70. Chomyn A, Martinuzzi A, Yoneda M, Daga A, Hurko O, Johns D, et al. MELAS mutation in mtDNA binding site for transcription termination factor causes defects in protein synthesis and in respiration but no change in levels of upstream and downstream mature transcripts. Proc Natl Acad Sci USA 89:4221–4225, 1992.

71. Obermaier-Kusser B, Paetzke-Brunner I, Enter C, Muller-Hocker J, Zierz S, Ruiten-

beek W, et al. Respiratory chain activity in tissues from patients (MELAS) with a point mutation of the mitochondrial genome [tRNA(Leu(UUR))]. FEBS Lett 286:67–70, 1991.

72. Ciafaloni E, Ricci E, Servidei S, Shanske S, Silvestri G, Manfredi G, et al. Widespread tissue distribution of a tRNALeu(UUR) mutation in the mitochondrial DNA of a patient with MELAS syndrome. Neurology 41:1663–1664, 1991.

73. Shoffner JM, Lott MT, Wallace DC. MERRF—a model disease for understanding the principles of mitochondrial genetics. Rev Neurol (Paris) 147(6–7):431–435, 1991.

74. Shoffner JM, Lott MT, Lezza AM, Seibel P, Ballinger SW, Wallace DC. Myoclonic epilepsy and ragged-red fiber disease (MERRF) is associated with a mitochondrial DNA tRNA(Lys) mutation. Cell 61:931–937, 1990.

75. Noer AS, Sudoyo H, Lertrit P, Thyagarajan D, Utthanaphol P, Kapsa R, et al. A tRNA(Lys) mutation in the mtDNA is the causal genetic lesion underlying myoclonic epilepsy and ragged-red fiber (MERRF) syndrome. Am J Hum Genet 49:715–722, 1991.

76. Byrne E, Trounce I, Marzuki S, Dennett X, Berkovic SF, Davis S, et al. Functional respiratory chain studies in mitochondrial cytopathies. Support for mitochondrial DNA heteroplasmy in myoclonus epilepsy and ragged red fibers (MERRF) syndrome. Acta Neuropathol Berl 81:318–323, 1991.

77. Seibel P, Degoul F, Bonne G, Romero N, Francois D, Paturneau Jouas M, et al. Genetic biochemical and pathophysiological characterization of a familial mitochondrial encephalomyopathy (MERRF). J Neurol Sci 105:217–224, 1991.

78. Shoffner JM, Wallace DC. Oxidative phosphorylation diseases. Disorders of two genomes. Adv Hum Genet 19:267–330, 1990.

79. Zeviani M, Gellera C, Antozzi C, Rimoldi M, Morandi L, Villani F, et al. Maternally inherited myopathy and cardiomyopathy: association with mutation in mitochondrial DNA tRNA(Leu)(UUR). Lancet 338:143–147, 1991.

80. Tanaka M, Ino H, Ohno K, Hattori K, Sato W. Mitochondrial mutation in fatal infantile myopathy. Lancet 336:1452, 1990.

81. Brown MD, Torroni A, Shoffner JM, Wallace DC. Mitochondrial tRNA(Thr) mutations and lethal infantile mitochondrial myopathy. Am J Hum Genet 51:446–447, 1992.

82. Mehta AB, Vulliamy T, Gordon Smith EC, Luzzatto L. A new genetic polymorphism in the 16S ribosomal RNA gene of human mitochondrial DNA. Ann Hum Genet 53:303–310, 1989.

83. Howell N, Lee A. Sequence analysis of mouse mitochondrial chloramphenicol-resistant mutants. Somat Cell Mol Genet 15:237–244, 1989.

84. Nagao T, Mauer AM. Concordance for drug-induced aplastic anemia in identical twins. N Engl J Med 281:7–11, 1969.

85. Rosenthal RL, Blackman A. Bone marrow hypoplasia following use of chloramphenicol eye drops. JAMA 191:136–137, 1965.

86. Howell A, Andrews TM, Watts RWE. Bone marrow cells resistant to chloramphenicol in chloramphenicol-induced aplastic anemia. Lancet II:81–82, 1975.

87. Zhang Q-H, Yan J-H, Ding Y-Q, Wong H. Genetic aspects of antibiotic induced deafness: mitochondrial inheritance. J Med Genet 28:79–83, 1991.

88. Jaber L, Shohat M, Bu X, Fischel Ghodsian N, Yang HY, Wang SJ, et al. Sensorineural deafness inherited as a tissue specific mitochondrial disorder. J Med Genet 29:86–90, 1992.

89. Harding AE, Hammans SR. Deletions of the mitochondrial genome. J Inherit Metab Dis 15:480–486, 1992.

90. Shoffner JM, Lott MT, Voljavec AS, Soueidan SA, Costigan DA, Wallace DC. Spontaneous Kearns-Sayre/chronic external ophthalmoplegia plus syndrome associated with a mitochondrial DNA deletion: a slip-replication model and metabolic therapy. Proc Natl Acad Sci USA 86:7952–7956, 1989.

91. Shanske S, Moraes CT, Lombes A, Miranda AF, Bonilla E, Lewis P, et al. Widespread tissue distribution of mitochondrial DNA deletions in Kearns-Sayre syndrome. Neurology 40:24–28, 1990.

92. Nakase H, Moraes CT, Rizzuto R, Lombes A, Dimauro S, Schon EA. Transcription and translation of deleted mitochondrial genomes in Kearns-Sayre syndrome: implications for pathogenesis. Am J Hum Genet 46:418–427, 1990.

93. Moraes CT, Dimauro S, Zeviani M, Lombes A, Shanske S, Miranda AF, et al. Mitochondrial DNA deletions in progressive external ophthalmoplegia and Kearns-Sayre syndrome. N Engl J Med 320:1293–1299, 1989.

94. Zeviani M, Moraes CT, Dimauro S, Nakase H, Bonilla E, Schon EA, et al. Deletions of mitochondrial DNA in Kearns-Sayre syndrome. Neurology 38:1339–1346, 1988.

95. Degoul F, Nelson I, Lestienne P, Francois D, Romero N, Duboc D, et al. Deletions of mitochondrial DNA in Kearns-Sayre syndrome and ocular myopathies: genetic, biochemical and morphological studies. J Neurol Sci 101:168–177, 1991.

96. Harding AE, Holt IJ, Cooper JM, Schapira AH, Sweeney M, Clark JB, et al. Mitochondrial myopathies: genetic defects. Biochem Soc Trans 18:519–522, 1990.

97. Lestienne P, Ponsot G. Kearns-Sayre syndrome with muscle mitochondrial DNA deletion letter. Lancet 1:885, 1988.

98. Zeviani M, Bresolin N, Gellera C, Bordoni A, Pannacci M, Amati P, et al. Nucleus-driven multiple large-scale deletions of the human mitochondrial genome: a new autosomal dominant disease. Am J Hum Genet 47:904–914, 1990.

99. Romero NB, Lestienne P, Marsac C, Paturneau Jouas M, Nelson I, Francois D, et al. Immunocytological and histochemical correlation in Kearns-Sayre syndrome with mtDNA deletion and partial cytochrome C oxidase deficiency in skeletal muscle. J Neurol Sci 93:297–309, 1989.

100. Rowland LP, Blake DM, Hirano M, Di Mauro S, Schon EA, Hays AP, et al. Clinical syndromes associated with ragged red fibers. Rev Neurol (Paris) 147:467–473, 1991.

101. Reichmann H, Degoul F, Gold R, Meurers B, Ketelsen UP, Hartmann J, et al. Histological, enzymatic and mitochondrial DNA studies in patients with Kearns-Sayre syndrome and chronic progressive external ophthalmoplegia. Eur Neurol 31:108–113, 1991.

102. Rowland LP, Blake DM, Hirano M, Di-Mauro S, Schon EA, Hays AP, et al. Clinical syndromes associated with ragged red fibers. Rev Neurol (Paris) 147(6–7):467–473, 1991.

103. Rotig A, Colonna M, Bonnefont JP, Blanche S, Fischer A, Saudubray JM, et al. Mitochondrial DNA deletion in Pearson's marrow/pancreas syndrome letter; comment. Lancet 1:902–903, 1989.

104. McShane MA, Hammans SR, Sweeney M, Holt IJ, Beattie TJ, Brett EM, et al. Pearson syndrome and mitochondrial encephalomyopathy in a patient with a deletion of mtDNA. Am J Hum Genet 48:39–42, 1991.

105. Yamadori I, Kurose A, Kobayashi S, Ohmori M, Imai T. Brain lesions of the Leigh-type distribution associated with a mitochondriopathy of Pearson's syndrome: light and electron microscopic study. Acta Neuropathol (Berl) 84:337–341, 1992.

106. Poulton J, Deadman ME, Gardiner RM. Tandem direct duplications of mitochondrial DNA in mitochondrial myopathy: analysis of nucleotide sequence and tissue distribution. Nucleic Acids Res 17:10223–10229, 1989.

107. Poulton J, Deadman ME, Gardiner RM. Duplications of mitochondrial DNA in mitochondrial myopathy. Lancet 1:236–240, 1989.

108. Poulton J. Duplications of mitochondrial DNA: implications for pathogenesis. J Inherit Metab Dis 15:487–498, 1992.

109. Zeviani M, Servidei S, Gellera C, Bertini E, Dimauro S, DiDonato S. An autosomal dominant disorder with multiple deletions of mitochondrial DNA starting at the D-loop region. Nature 339:309–311, 1989.

110. Servidei S, Zeviani M, Manfredi G, Ricci E, Silvestri G, Bertini E, et al. Dominantly inherited mitochondrial myopathy with multiple deletions of mitochondrial DNA: clinical, morphologic, and biochemical studies. Neurology 41:1053–1059, 1991.

111. Zeviani M. Nucleus-driven mutations of human mitochondrial DNA. J Inherit Metab Dis 15:456–471, 1992.

112. Trounce I, Byrne E, Marzuki S. Decline in skeletal muscle mitochondrial respiratory chain function: possible factor in ageing. Lancet 1:637–639, 1989.

113. Wallace DC. Mitochondrial genetics: a paradigm for aging and degenerative diseases? Science 256:628–632, 1992.

114. Hattori K, Tanaka M, Sugiyama S, Obayashi T, Ito T, Satake T, et al. Age-dependent increase in deleted mitochondrial DNA in the human heart: possible contributory factor to presbycardia. Am Heart J 121:1735–1742, 1991.

115. Sugiyama S, Hattori K, Hayakawa M, Ozawa T. Quantitative analysis of age-associated accumulation of mitochondrial DNA with deletion in human hearts. Biochem Biophys Res Commun 180:894–899, 1991.

116. Cortopassi GA, Arnheim N. Detection of a specific mitochondrial DNA deletion in tissues of older humans. Nucleic Acids Res 18:6927–6933, 1990.

117. Corral-Debrinski M, Shoffner JM, Lott MT, Wallace DC. Association of mitochondrial DNA damage with aging and coronary atherosclerotic heart disease. Mutat Res 275:169–180, 1992.

118. Hattori K, Ogawa T, Kondo T, Mochizuki M, Tanaka M, Sugiyama S, et al. Cardiomyopathy with mitochondrial DNA mutations. Am Heart J 122:866–869, 1991.

119. Ozawa T, Tanaka M, Sugiyama S, Hattori K, Ito T, Ohno K, et al. Multiple mitochondrial DNA deletions exist in cardiomyocytes of patients with hypertrophic or dilated cardiomyopathy. Biochem Biophys Res Commun 170:830–836, 1990.

120. Corral-Debrinski M, Stepien G, Shoffner JM, Lott MT, Kanter K, Wallace DC. Hypoxemia is associated with mitochondrial DNA damage and gene induction. Implications for cardiac disease. JAMA 266:1812–1816, 1991.

121. Kadenbach B, Muller-Hocker J. Mutations of mitochondrial DNA and human death. Naturwissenschaften 77:221–225, 1990.

122. Parker WD, Jr., Boyson SJ, Parks JK. Abnormalities of the electron transport chain in idiopathic Parkinson's disease. Ann Neurol 26:719–723, 1989.

123. Bindoff LA, Birch Machin M, Cartlidge NE, Parker WD, Jr., Turnbull DM. Mitochondrial function in Parkinson's disease. Lancet 2:49, 1989.

124. Schapira AH, Cooper JM, Dexter D, Jenner P, Clark JB, Marsden CD. Mitochondrial complex I deficiency in Parkinson's disease. Lancet 1:1269, 1989.

125. Bindoff LA, Birch Machin MA, Cartlidge NE, Parker WD, Turnbull DM. Respiratory chain abnormalities in skeletal muscle from patients with Parkinson's disease. J Neurol Sci 104:203–208, 1991.

126. Dagani F, Anderson JJ, Chase TN. Mitochondrial function in Parkinson's disease. Ann Neurol 32:226–227, 1992.

127. Wallace DC, Shoffner JM, Watts RL, Juncos JL, Torroni A. Mitochondrial oxidative phosphorylation defects in Parkinson's disease. Ann Neurol 32:113–114, 1992.

128. Shoffner JM, Watts RL, Juncos JL, Torroni A, Wallace DC. Mitochondrial oxidative-phosphorylation defects in Parkinson's disease. Ann Neurol 30(3):332–339, 1991.

129. Di Monte DA. Mitochondrial DNA and Parkinson's disease. Neurology 41:38–42, 1991.

130. Ozawa T, Tanaka M, Ino H, Ohno K, Sano T, Wada Y, et al. Distinct clustering of point mutations in mitochondrial DNA among patients with mitochondrial encephalomyopathies and with Parkinson's disease. Biochem Biophys Res Commun 176:938–946, 1991.

131. Lestienne P, Nelson I, Riederer P, Reichmann H, Jellinger K. Mitochondrial DNA in postmortem brain from patients with Parkinson's disease. J Neurochem 56:1819, 1991.

132. Lesteinne P, Nelson J, Riederer P, Jellinger K, Reichmann H. Normal mitochondrial genome in brain from patients with Parkinson's disease and complex I defect. J Neurochem 55:1810–1812, 1990.

133. Kopin IJ. MPTP: an industrial chemical and contaminant of illicit narcotics stimulates a new era in research on Parkinson's disease. Environ Health Perspect 75:45–51, 1987.

134. Lin FH, Lin R, Wisniewski HM, Hwang YW, Grundke Iqbal I, Healy Louie G, et al. Detection of point mutations in codon 331 of mitochondrial NADH dehydrogenase subunit 2 in Alzheimer's brains. Biochem Biophys Res Commun 182:238–246, 1992.

135. Petruzzella V, Chen X, Schon EA. Is a point mutation in the mitochondrial ND2 gene associated with Alzheimer's disease. Biochem Biophys Res Commun 186:491–497, 1992.

7

Genomic Imprinting

Certain genes demonstrate a parent-of-origin effect in their expression. This parent-of-origin effect occurs because these genes are modified during their transmission via oocytes or spermatocytes. The process of germ cell-specific modification of a gene is known as *genomic imprinting,* a term that was coined by Helen Crouse. In 1960, she described the phenomenon in this way.

A chromosome which passes through the male germ line will acquire an "imprint" which will result in behavior exactly opposite to the "imprint" conferred of the same chromosome by the female germ line. In other words, the "imprint" a chromosome bears is unrelated to the genic constitution of the chromosome and is determined only by the sex of the germ line through which the chromosome has been inherited.[1]

In its brief history, the study of genomic imprinting has had three phases. In the first, it was demonstrated that the maternal and paternal genomes do not make equivalent contributions to mammalian development. In the second phase, it was demonstrated that imprinting is confined to certain regions of the genome and the delineation of those regions. Within those regions, some genes may show a maternal imprint, whereas others show a paternal imprint. The third phase has been concerned with the identification of the molecular mechanisms of genomic imprinting.

EVIDENCE FOR GENOMIC IMPRINTING

The first evidence in mammals for a nonequivalent contribution from maternal and paternal genomes came from the genetic analysis of ovarian teratomas and hydatidiform moles, conditions of aberrant embryonic development (Table 7.1). Further evidence was provided from experimental efforts aimed at inducing

Table 7.1. Evidence for genomic imprinting

Condition	Chromosomal constitution	Parental origin
Human		
Ovarian teratoma[2,3]	46,XX	Maternal
Hydatidiform mole[4]	46,XX or 46,XY	Paternal
Partial mole	69,XXX, 69,XXY or 69,XYY	Paternal
Severe growth retardation with fibrotic placenta [5,6]	69,XXX or 69,XXY	Maternal
Mouse		
Gynogenote [7–12]	20,XX	Maternal
Androgenote[10,12]	20,XX or 20,XY	Paternal

development from zygotes that contained two maternally derived or two paternally derived pronuclei.

Ovarian teratomas. The first indication of genomic imprinting in humans came from the study of ovarian teratomas. These tumors differentiate to contain somatic, but not placental, elements. All ovarian teratomas have a 46,XX chromosomal constitution.[2] As judged by the homozygosity of centromeric chromosomal polymorphisms, the tumors originate from germ cells after the first meiotic division.[3] Diploidy was achieved by suppression of the second meiotic division or by fusion of the second polar body with the oocyte. Thus, these studies suggested that these tumors develop in the absence of a paternally derived genome.

Hydatidiform moles. Hydatidiform moles are gestational trophoblastic tumors. These can be divided into complete moles that affect the whole conceptus and partial moles that show evidence of a fetus in addition to the trophoblast.[13] On the basis of chromosomal polymorphism analysis, seven complete hydatidiform moles were shown to contain chromosomes that were paternal in origin.[4] These findings could be explained on the basis of fertilization of an enucleated oocyte with a diploid sperm, with two haploid sperm, or with one haploid sperm that underwent endoreduplication.

All partial moles have a triploid chromosomal constitution; the extra set is paternal in origin.[5,6] By contrast, triploid conceptions with an extra set of maternal chromosomes do not have molar changes. Rather, the fetal development is severely retarded, the extraembryonic membranes are sparse, and the placenta is small and fibrotic.[14,15] These observations suggest that paternally derived genes play a critical role in the development and maintenance of the extraembryonic membranes and placenta and that maternally derived genes play a critical role in the development of the fetus.

Experimental gynogenotes and androgenotes. Mouse embryos have been constructed experimentally that contain two copies of the maternal genome and no copies of the paternal genome *(gynogenotes)*. Gynogenotes have been induced by parthenogenesis or by experimental manipulation of the nuclei in one-cell embryos. Parthenogenesis has been induced by ethanol exposure of oocytes, which caused fusion of the second polar body with the oocyte, failure of cleavage of the second polar body with fusion of the oocyte and polar body pronuclei, or formation of a single pronucleus during metaphase II that contained a duplicated set of chromosomes.[7–9] Alternatively, gynogenotes have been created by injection of the female pronucleus into oocytes in one-cell embryos. [10–12] These parthenogenic or gynogenic embryos differentiated to the morula or blastula stage and initiated implantation but failed to develop normal extraembryonic membranes. One explanation for this finding was the presence of homozygous lethal genes in the embryo. This hypothesis was ruled out by introducing a female pronucleus from a different inbred strain into a fertilized oocyte from which the male pronucleus was removed.[10] The embryos all died within a few days of implantation. By contrast, introduction of a male pronucleus from the same inbred strains into the oocyte resulted in normal embryonic development, thus ruling against recessive genes.[9,16] These experiments demonstrate the requirement for a paternal contribution for the development of normal extraembryonic structures.

Androgenotes were created by extraction of the maternal pronucleus from the zygote and introduction of a second male pronucleus.[10,12] Most (75%) of these embryos developed to the blastocyst stage. Those with a YY chromosomal constitution did not. A small number of embryos implanted when transferred to a foster mother and these contained only extraembryonic components. This experimental condition demonstrated the need for a maternal contribution for normal embryonic development.

CHROMOSOMAL REGIONS DEMONSTRATING GENOMIC IMPRINTING

Uniparental disomy in mice. To localize regions in the mouse that are subject to chromosomal imprinting, mice were bred with two copies of specific chromosomes or chromosomal regions from one parent and none from the other [17]—that is, they had uniparental disomy. The mice were created by breeding parents with Robertsonian translocations. All mouse chromosomes are acrocentric, so fusion of any two chromosomes at the centromere produces Robertsonian translocations. In mice that are balanced for these translocations, nondisjunction occurs at meiosis, so some gametes are disomic for a particular chromosome, whereas others are nullisomic, and the remainder of the chromosomes segregate normally (Fig. 7.1). When two mice that have the same Robertsonian translocation are crossed, a proportion of the zygotes are formed by fusion of a gamete that contains both homologues of a particular chromosome to a gamete that does not contain any homologues. The offspring have balanced chromosomal constitutions with uniparental disomy for the particular chromosome.

To further refine the region that affects the phenotype of the mice, parents have been bred who had balanced reciprocal translocations between nonhomologous chromosomes. This has led to offspring who had uniparental disomy for

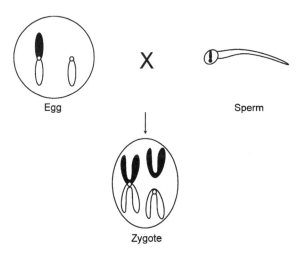

Figure 7.1. Breeding for maternal uniparental disomy in mice with Robertsonian translocations.

a particular region. These mice had maternal or paternal duplication of the region with corresponding paternal or maternal deficiency for that region. Zygotes with maternal or paternal disomy for chromosomes 1, 4, 5, 9, 13, 14, and 15 survived normally.[17,18] Two parental origin effects were observed for other chromosomes, lethality and development of abnormal phenotypes (Table 7.2). For example, maternal disomy for chromosome 6 is lethal, whereas paternal disomy for chromosome 6 is associated with normal development. Lethality has also been observed for maternal uniparental disomy for chromosomes 2, 7, and 8, and paternal uniparental disomy for distal chromosome 7.[19] Uniparental disomy for other regions has led to behavioral and physical abnormalities. For example, maternal disomy for distal chromosome 2 was associated with hypo-

Table 7.2. Mouse chromosomal regions demonstrating parental origin effects[19]

Region	Maternal disomy	Paternal disomy
Proximal 2	Lethal	Normal
Distal 2	Hypokinetic	Hyperkinetic, kinked tail
Proximal 6	Early lethal	Normal
Proximal 7	Neonatal lethal?	Normal
Distal 7	Early embryonic lethal	Mid-fetal lethal
Distal 8	Lethal	Normal
Proximal 11	Lethal	Lethal
Chromosome 17	Normal?	Maternal deletion associated with lethality (Tme)

kinetic behavior whereas paternal disomy was associated with hyperkinetic behavior and a kinked tail. These findings suggested that imprinted genes may be clustered in specific chromosomal regions.

The imprinting process may affect discreet loci on chromosomes rather than multiple loci within a region. Deletions of proximal chromosome 17 in the short tail or T complex region are lethal only when inherited from the mother.[20] The absence of a gene, Tme (for *maternal effect*), was postulated to result in embryonic death at day 15 of gestation. Four genes have been found in the deleted region: t-complex polypeptide-1 (Tcp1), plasminogen (Plg), superoxide dismutase-2 (Sod-2), and insulin-like growth factor type 2/mannose-6-phosphate receptor (Igf2r). Each of these genes was tested as a candidate for genomic imprinting by Northern blot analysis of heterozygous embryos that inherited the Tme deletion from either the mother or the father. Igf2r was found to be expressed when the deletion was inherited from the father, but not from the mother.[21] The three other genes were found to be expressed when the Tme deletion was inherited from either the mother or the father. This demonstrated that the maternal allele of Igf2r is imprinted. The Igf2 receptor binds the growth factor and, via mannose-6-phosphate residues, some 50 lysosomal enzymes.[22,23] When bound to the receptor, these enzymes are targeted to the lysosomes either for internalization or for degradation. Based on its location, expression, and physiological effects, deletion of the paternal Igf2r gene with resulting lack of expression of the maternal allele is associated with lethality.

The insulin-like growth factor, type 2 (Igf2) loci is also subject to genomic imprinting.[24] This was demonstrated first in "knock-out" experiments in transgenic mice,[25] in which the Igf2 locus was inactivated by homologous recombination of the wild type gene in embryonic stem cells to a Igf2 gene that was silenced by insertion of a sequence for neomycin resistance (neo). When transmitted in the heterozygous state, those mice inheriting a knock-out gene from the father were smaller than their littermates and remained about 40% smaller throughout their lifetimes. The phenotype of homozygous Igf2-deficient mice was the same as that of paternal heterozygotes. These heterozygous mice produced defective transcripts containing the inserted neo gene sequence, but no normal (maternal) transcript. These studies demonstrated that the genes for Igf2 and its receptor, Igf2r, are subject to genomic imprinting, albeit reciprocal, in their parent of origin.

The mouse H19 gene is subject to genomic imprinting, with the maternal, but not the paternal, copy being expressed.[26] This unusual gene encodes one of the most abundant transcripts in mouse embryos.[27] Initially expressed during the blastocyst stage of development, the RNA accumulates on 28s particles in the cytoplasm of tissues of endodermal and mesodermal origin. The RNA is transcribed using the enzyme RNA polymerase II, and it was spliced and polyadenylated. Despite sequence similarity between the mouse and human genes, they did not share an open reading frame. In fact, the absence of a long open reading frame suggested that this RNA may not encode a protein at all. Nonetheless, H19 serves an essential function. When the RNA was overexpressed in transgenic mice, the embryos died between day 14 and birth.[28]

Imprinted genes appear to be clustered on specific chromosomes (Table 7.3). The mouse H19 gene maps to the distal segment of chromosome 7 about 75–100 kb from the Igf2 gene;[29] however, the Igf2 gene demonstrates paternal imprinting, whereas the H19 gene demonstrates maternal. The linkage and imprinting effects of the Igf2 and H19 genes are conserved in humans with these genes mapping to 11p15.[30,31] Based on studies on the Beckwith-Wiedemann syndrome, these genes may share a common imprinting regulator (see below).

Disorders of human development. Two conditions, Prader-Willi syndrome and Angelman syndrome, share mental retardation as their only common feature. Patients with Prader-Willi syndrome have narrow bifrontal diameters, small hands and feet, hypogonadism, and a compulsion to eat.[40] By contrast, patients with Angelman syndrome have small heads with flat occiputs, happy dispositions, and marionette-like movements, thus causing this to be known originally as the "Happy Puppet syndrome."[41]

The first indication of a parental origin effect in Prader-Willi syndrome was the demonstration of deletions of the proximal long arm of chromosome 15 (Fig. 7.2).[42] In large series, deletions of chromosome 15 (15q11–13) have been found in 50–60% of cases of Prader-Willi syndrome. In all cases, the deletion was inherited from the father.[44,45] By contrast, deletions of chromosome 15 in the same region [del(15)(q11-q13)] were observed in 50–60% of patients with Angelman syndrome (Fig. 7.2).[46–49] In all of these cases, the deletions are inherited from the mother.

In 20–25% of cases of Prader-Willi syndrome uniparental disomy for mater-

Table 7.3. Genes demonstrating genomic imprinting

Gene	Human imprint	Human chromosomal location	Mouse imprint	Mouse chromosomal location
IGF2[21,29,31,32]	Maternal	11p15	Maternal	Distal 7
H19[29,30,32]	Paternal	11p15	Paternal	Distal 7
KIP2[33]	Paternal (partial)	11p15	n.d.	n.d.
Mash-2[34]	n.d.	n.d.	Paternal	Distal 7
Insulin-2[34]	—	No human homologue	Maternal	Distal 7
IGF2R[21]			Paternal	Proximal 17
SNRPN[35,36]	Maternal	15q11-q13	Maternal	Central 7
IPW[37]	Maternal	15q11-q13	n.d.	n.d.
ZNF127[38]	Maternal	15q11-q13	n.d.	Central 7
PAR1[39]	Maternal	15q11-q13	n.d.	n.d.
PAR5[39]	Maternal	15q11-q13	n.d.	n.d.

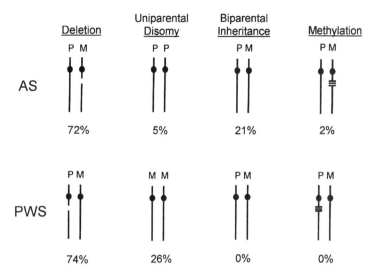

Figure 7.2. Molecular classes of chromosome 15 abnormalities in individuals with Angelman and Prader-Willi syndromes.[43]

nal chromosome 15 was present (Fig. 7.2).[50,51] This may be either isodisomy or heterodisomy. In about 5% of cases of Angelman syndrome, uniparental disomy for paternal chromosomes 15 was observed.[52,53] Some cases of Prader-Willi syndrome have been described that were compatible with somatic recombination of chromosome 15, resulting in paternal heterodisomy.[54] One family was described with occurrence of one case of Angelman syndrome and two cases of Prader-Willi syndrome in first cousins all having a unbalanced translocation, t(15;22)(q13•1). The inheritance of these disorders was compatible with the predicted parental origin effect. The development of these conditions resulted from transmission of the Robertsonian translocation followed by postzygotic nondisjunction. The women carrying the balanced translocation had a high risk of having children with Angelman syndrome whereas their brothers had a high risk of having children with Prader-Willi syndrome.[55] These studies have demonstrated that the proximal region of the long arm of chromosome 15 was subject to both maternal and paternal imprinting effects. The maternally imprinted segment was necessary to prevent Angelman syndrome, whereas the paternally imprinted segment was necessary to prevent Prader-Willi syndrome.[56]

Several maternally imprinted genes have been identified in the smallest genomic region deleted in individuals with Prader-Willi syndrome. These include SNRPN, a ribonuclear protein subunit thought to be involved in brain-specific RNA splicing; [35,36] IPW, an abundant noncoding RNA;[37] and ZNF127, a protein with a zinc finger motif that is presumed to bind nucleic acid.[38] Two other maternally imprinted genes, PAR1 and PAR5, have been identified in this region. To date, these genes have been less well characterized.[39] The gene product of SNRPN may not play a direct role in the development of the Prader-Willi phenotype. One patient with Prader-Willi syndrome had an unbalanced, paternally derived translocation with the breakpoint mapping between SNRPN and PAR1. The expression of the SNRPN gene was unaffected, whereas the IPW and PAR1 alleles were not expressed. These findings were consistent with the elimination of a *cis*-acting candidate imprinting center mapping proximal to SNRPN.[57]

The critical region for Angelman syndrome is distinct from that for Prader-Willi syndrome. In one family, three siblings affected with Angelman syndrome inherited the same small deletion of chromosome 15 from their unaffected mother. She, in turn, inherited it from her father. Had this critical region included genes for Prader-Willi syndrome, the mother should have been affected with the condition.[58] Recently, the UBE3/E6-AP was identified as a candidate for Angelman syndrome on the basis of de novo mutations in four cases and an inherited mutation in one family.[59,60] Remarkably, biallelic expression of this gene has been observed for most of the tissues tested so far. Maternal imprinting is confined to a brain-specific isoform.

Parent-of-origin methylation patterns for DNA markers in the q11-q13 region of chromosome 15 have been used to diagnose these conditions (Fig. 7.2).[38] Normal individuals demonstrate both maternal and paternal patterns. Prader-Willi syndrome cases that arise from deletion or from uniparental disomy show a maternal imprinting pattern for these markers. By contrast, the Angelman syndrome cases that arise from deletion or from uniparental disomy show a paternal imprinting pattern.

Not all cases of Angelman syndrome have been shown to arise from deletion or uniparental disomy. Approximately 20% of individuals with Angelman syndrome have biparental methylation patterns of markers on 15q11-q13 (Fig. 7.2). These cases are probably due to mutation in a single gene. Familial cases of Angelman syndrome are compatible with this hypothesis.[61]

Beckwith-Wiedemann syndrome is a condition associated with somatic overgrowth (macroglossia, exomphalos, visceromegaly, gigantism, and islet cell hyperplasia) and a predisposition to tumor development, including Wilms tumor, rhabdomyosarcoma, hepatoblastoma, and adrenocortical carcinoma.[62–64] Several genetic mechanisms have been associated with the development of this condition which have demonstrated that unlike Prader-Willi and Angelman syndromes, Beckwith-Wiedemann syndrome results from overexpression of the unimprinted allele of an imprinted gene. Duplication of the short arm of chromosome 11 (11p15) has been demonstrated in some sporadic cases. In each of these cases, the duplicated segment was of paternal origin.[65,66] Other sporadic cases were associated with paternal isodisomy for chromosomal markers that map to 11p15.[67–69] Familial cases of Beckwith-Wiedemann syndrome have been described, demonstrating vertical transmission. In these families the development of the condition was linked tightly to genetic markers at 11p15.[70–72] In almost every case, children developed the condition only if the mutation were inherited through the mother, despite the fact that some of the carrier mothers showed no signs of this condition.[73] This suggests that the mutation inactivates an "imprinting" locus in the mother, resulting in its failure to imprint the maternal alleles of the locus at 11p15. This failure to imprint leads to biallelic expression (and hence, overexpression) of the Beckwith-Wiedemann syndrome–causing locus.

The disomic segment in individuals with Beckwith-Wiedemann syndrome and uniparental disomy includes the imprinted gene, IGF2.[30,31] IGF2 is a major growth factor in humans and has been proposed as a candidate for this syndrome. The cases of paternally derived duplication of 11p15 and paternal uniparental disomy are consistent with expression of this gene. The familial cases which are preferentially transmitted by carrier mothers are consistent with loss of the maternal imprint at this locus. The finding of biallelic expression of IGF2 locus in cases of Beckwith-Wiedemann syndrome that were not associated with paternal disomy or chromosomal duplication demonstrated disruption of imprinting of the IGF2 locus.[74] As noted earlier, the mouse Igf2 gene is imprinted and only the paternal allele is transcribed.[24] Chimeric mice that contained a duplicated segment for distal paternal chromosome 7, including the Igf2 gene, had growth enhancement similar to that which is observed in Beckwith-Wiedemann syndrome.[75]

Cancer syndromes associated with genomic imprinting. A subset of individuals with Beckwith-Wiedemann syndrome (5–10%) develop Wilms tumor, adrenocortical carcinoma, hepatoblastoma, or embryonal rhabdomyosarcoma.[64] Structural or transmission abnormalities involving chromosome 11 suggest a shared genetic basis for the development of Beckwith-Wiedemann syndrome and these tumors. Sporadic cases of Wilms tumor have been associated with deletion of DNA markers on the short arm of chromosome 11 in the q13-q15 region.[76] In greater than 90% of sporadic cases associated with deletion, the loss of alleles occurred on the maternally derived chromosome.[77,78] Richard Wilkens interpreted this to mean that the paternal allele was imprinted and functionally inactive and that deletion of the maternal chromosome 11 resulted in loss of a tumor suppressor gene and hence tumor development.[79]

The WT1 gene is located at 11p13 and has been shown not to be imprinted. Detailed analysis of sporadic cases of Wilms tumor identified a subset with loss of heterozygosity that was confined to distal chromosome 11 at band p15.[72,80] Thus, these studies demonstrated a second locus for Wilms tumor at 11p15 distinct from the WT1 gene at 11p13. Mitotic recombination mapping also localized the gene for embryonal rhabdomyosarcoma to 11p15.[81] The existence of a second Wilms tumor gene, WT2, has been confirmed by familial cases of Wilms tumor in which linkage was demonstrated to genetic markers at 11p15.[70–72] Thus, loss of maternal alleles at 11p15 may act as the second hit for the development of embryonal tumors associated with Beckwith-Wiedemann syndrome.[67,68,82]

Several genes that map to 11p15, including IGF2, H19, and KIP2, demonstrate genomic imprinting in human kidneys, albeit incomplete for KIP2, and thus are candidates for the WT2 gene.[31,33,82] In cases of Wilms tumor without loss of heterozygosity, the imprinting of IGF2 and H19 is erased so that there is biallelic expression of IGF2 and reduced expression of the unimprinted H19 and KIP2 alleles. These findings are compatible with roles for IGF2 as a dominant oncogene and for H19 and KIP2 as tumor suppressor genes.[84–89] Further evidence supporting a role for H19 as a tumor suppressor gene was the observation that growth retardation occurred in two embryonal tumor cell lines when transfected with H19. Tumorigenicity was likewise interrupted when the transfected cells were injected into nude mice.[90]

Parental origin effects have been observed for hereditary glomus tumors.[91] Hereditary glomus tumors, or paragangliomas, are benign, slowly growing masses in the head or neck. Half of the cases are familial. The sex of the transmitting parent determines whether individuals who inherit the disease gene are affected. All affected individuals who have been studied to date inherited their disease genes from their fathers. The phenotype is not expressed in the offspring of an affected female until transmitted through a male carrier. These observations are compatible with genomic imprinting. The gene for this condition has been mapped to 11q23 on the basis of linkage analysis.[92]

MECHANISMS OF IMPRINTING IN MAMMALS

Methylation. Both methylation of DNA and the timing of DNA replication are markers for genomic imprinting. Cytosine residues in DNA are methylated at the 5' position of CG dinucleotides.[93] Cytosine methylation is a stable epigenetic change that correlates with the expression of genes.[93–95] The state of methylation of CG dinucleotides can be readily assayed.[93,96]

Transgenes were the first genetic markers that were shown to have differential parent-of-origin methylation. Randomly inserted into one or more chromosomes, the structure and expression of transgenes were affected by the chromosomal position. The effect of parental origin on methylation and expression as tested in animals that were heterozygous for single insertions of the transgenes. These animals were bred and their offspring were tested for imprinting effects for modification of the DNA and expression of the transgene.[97,98] For SV CAT IgH,[98] troponin I (TNI),[99] and RSV Ig c-myc,[100,101] the pattern of methylation in somatic cells was determined by the parent of origin. The transgenes were undermethylated if transmitted from the father and highly methylated if transmitted by the mother. Depending on the gamete of origin, the pattern of methylation was either the same or altered in the subsequent generation. The effects appeared to have been independent of the sequence, the copy number, and the size (3–20 kb) of the transgene. In one case, a human hepatitis B surface antigen (HBsAg) transgene became irreversibly methylated when transmitted through a maternal germ line.[102]

To understand when these methylation differences occurred, a developmental study was undertaken with the RSV Ig c-myc transgene.[101] On day 13.5 of development, the transgene was unmethylated in germ cells regardless of the sex of the embryo or of the sex of the parent from whom the transgene was inherited. This suggested that the methylation patterns were erased in early germ cells. By day 17.5, a new methylation pattern was observed in male germ cells, during the stage of spermatogonial proliferation. A similar pattern was observed in the testis of newborn mice. The pattern of methylation in pachytene spermatocytes and round spermatids was the same as that in mature sperm, suggesting that methylation occurred during meiosis and/or spermiogenesis. In female germ cells, the unmethylated pattern was observed at 17.5 days and at birth (when oocytes are arrested in the dictyotene stage of meiosis I). Mature, unfertilized eggs showed a different pattern, suggesting that the methylation occurred between meiosis I and ovulation.

The paternally inherited transgene underwent further modification after fertilization in the zygote.[101] The methylation was lost in both the inner cell mass and the trophectoderm of the blastocyst at 3.5 days of development. The adult pattern of methylation was observed in postimplantation embryos at 6.5 days in both embryonic and extraembryonic tissues. By contrast, the maternally transmitted transgene did not undergo further modification after fertilization. The expression of the RSV Ig c-myc transgene was affected by the parental origin—that is, the gene was expressed only when transmitted by the father and not by the mother. The expression correlated with the hypomethylation of paternally derived DNA.

Methylation of the Igf2 and Igf2r genes has also been examined for a parental origin effect at different stages of development. A CG island on the 5' side of the Igf2 gene that comprises one of the two strong promoters is unmethylated at both parental alleles.[103] By contrast, differences in methylation were observed in a region several kilobases upstream. The site on the paternal chromosome was more methylated and correlated with expression of the Igf2 gene. The allele-specific methylation pattern was established during embryogenesis after the blastula stage.

Two methylated regions demonstrating a parent-of-origin effect were demonstrated for the Igf2r gene.[104] Region I contained the transcription initiation site and was methylated only on the silent paternal chromosome. This methylation was acquired after fertilization. Region 2 was located in an intron and was methylated only on the expressed maternal chromosome. Methylation of this region was inherited in a stable fashion from the oocyte. These studies suggested that modification of only a few residues in DNA may be necessary for maintaining parental identity during development.

To further examine the role of methylation in imprinting, the cytosine-5-methyltransferase gene was knocked out by homologous recombination in embryonic stem (ES) cells.[105] This mutation did not alter the viability or proliferation of ES cells in culture. When the mutation was introduced into the germ line of mice, it caused a recessive, lethal phenotype. The homologous mice were small, had delayed development, and did not survive past midgestation. The normally silent paternal H19 allele was activated. By contrast, the active paternal Igf2 allele and maternal Igf2r allele were repressed. These studies demonstrated that methylation of these genes is required for normal imprinting and development to occur.

Asynchronous replication. Another mechanism that is associated with genomic imprinting is the time during the cell cycle when genes are replicated.[106,107] Non-imprinted housekeeping genes are replicated early in S phase. Tissue-specific genes are expressed early in S phase in the tissues in which they are expressed and late in tissues in which they are not expressed. The active X chromosome replicates early, whereas the inactive X chromosome replicates late.

The imprinted genes, IGF2, H19, IGF2R, and SNRPN in humans and mice, have replication asynchrony between the two alleles. The paternal allele always replicated early despite the fact that only the maternal H19 and IGF2R alleles are expressed in humans and mice. The imprinted genes are embedded in large DNA domains whose replication timing is regulated differently on the two chromosomes. Nonimprinted genes within these domains, such as GABRB3 on human chromosome 15 and insulin II on mouse chromosome 7, show the same asynchronous replication as the imprinted genes with these chromosomal domains. These studies demonstrate that asynchronous replication is a marker for the domains in which imprinted genes reside. Other factors determine whether they are maternally or paternally imprinted, or not at all.

CONSEQUENCES OF GENOMIC IMPRINTING

Epistasis. Genomic imprinting is a mechanism for regulating gene expression. This requires the presence of two distinct loci, one that is imprinted and the other that is imprinting. This ability of one gene to functionally inactivate another is an example of a modifying gene that demonstrates a gamete-of-origin effect.[108] The imprinting locus may be polymorphic in its effect on the target locus, resulting in complete or partial inactivation or no inactivation at all. The resulting activity of the imprinted locus determines whether the phenotype that it encodes is expressed in a dominant or recessive fashion. When one of the alleles is completely inactivated by the imprinting gene, the phenotype is expressed in a dominant fashion. When it is inactivated in some cells, but not in others, the phenotype is dominant, but with variable expressivity. When the target allele is not inactivated (or the imprint is erased), the phenotype is expressed in a recessive way.

Imprinting loci may act in *cis,* inactivating adjacent loci, or in *trans.* An analogous case of the *cis* effect is that of X chromosome inactivation. *Cis* inactivation by an imprinting locus would occur over a shorter region.[107] This would be recognized as a contiguous gene syndrome with a parent-of-origin effect. Beckwith-Wiedemann syndrome with Wilms tumor fits such a model. An imprinting locus acting in *trans* could cause multiple variably expressed and nonsyntenic phenotypes in an individual or among the individuals within a family. The disorders are nonsyntenic because loci on more than one chromosome may be affected by the activity of the dominance modifier.

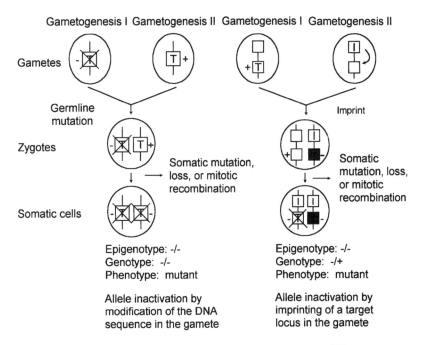

Figure 7.3. Mechanisms of allele inactivation in human cancers.[109]

Genomic imprinting provides an alternative model to the two-hit hypothesis of carcinogenesis originally developed by Knudson (Fig. 7.3).[109] In this model there is a major regulatory/suppressor gene for which loss of heterozygosity is associated with tumor development. The genetic hits that inactivate this locus may be of two types, allele inactivation by modification of the nucleotide sequence and allele inactivation by genomic imprinting. In the first type, inheritance of the disease is linked to markers on the chromosome that carries the tumor suppressor allele. The sex of the parent transmitting the disease allele does not have an effect. In the second type, the inactivation of the allele is not dependent on the allele itself but on the *trans*-acting effect of an imprinting gene. This gene need not be linked to the tumor suppressor locus. The activity of the imprinting gene may be reversible, thus accounting for spontaneous regression or mixed normal and malignant cell histology in some tumors. This model can explain a familial basis for certain tumors for which several different loci have been identified. This model can be tested by demonstrating parental origin effects for one or more genetic markers.

Carmen Sapienza has suggested that familial cancer syndromes with mixed tumors may represent an example of a *trans*-acting imprinting locus.[109] The general cancer syndrome may appear to be acting as a dominant, but different individuals within a family may be affected with different primary tumors, depending on the cell type in which the second genetic hit occurred.

CRITERIA FOR DEMONSTRATING GENOMIC IMPRINTING

Genomic imprinting has often been confused with other genetic mechanisms that show a gamete-of-origin effect. There are several criteria that may aid in this distinction. First, uniparental disomy or deletions with an invariant parent-of-origin effect should be identified in some sporadic cases. Second, a genetic marker (e.g., methylation of cytosine residues) should correlate with the parent-of-origin effect on the allele in question. This event should remain the same when transmitted through a gamete of the same type and should be altered when transmitted through an allele of the opposite type. Third, the imprinting locus should usually map to a different site from the imprinted locus. For mapping purposes, the imprinting locus is informative only in those gametes that show a parent-of-origin effect. Fourth, allelic variation in the imprinting locus should correlate with allelic variation in the imprinted locus. Inactivation of the imprinting locus should be correlated with activation of the imprinted locus.

These assumptions are based on a model of genomic imprinting in which there is relative or complete inactivation of a given allele. This model accounts for the development of phenotypes that are sensitive to gene dosage. An alternative model of genomic imprinting is that the expression of the two alleles is different, so different products are made. There are two consequences to this form of imprinting. If the two alleles complement one another, the expression of the phenotype may be dependent on the genotype of each allele. If the products of the two alleles do not complement one another, two different phenotypes may map to the locus, each showing a parent-of-origin effect. Although such an effect has not yet been observed in mammalian systems, the mating type locus in *Saccharomyces cerevisiae* remains heterozygous in isogenic diploid strains. Different gene products are produced from the two alleles at this locus. These act in *cis* to regulate themselves and in *trans* on other loci that are involved in gametogenesis.[110]

Genomic imprinting highlights one of the ways that genes are processed differentially in oocytes and spermatocytes. The faithfulness of replication of certain genes can vary between the two types of germ cells. When the rate of mutation is accelerated in one germ cell type, the resulting phenotype can show a parent-of-origin effect in its transmission.

REFERENCES

1. Crouse HV. The controlling element in sex chromosome behavior in sciara. Genetics 45:1429–1443, 1960.
2. Galton M, Benirschke K. Forty-six chromosomes in an ovarian teratoma. Lancet 2:761–762, 1959.
3. Linder D, McCaw BK, Hecht F. Parthenogenic origin of benign ovarian teratomas. N Engl J Med 292:63–66, 1975.
4. Lawler SD, Povey S, Fisher RA, Pickthall VJ. Genetic studies on hydatidiform moles. II.The origin of complete moles. Ann Hum Genet 46:209–222, 1982.

5. Kaufman MH, Lee KK, Speirs S. Influence of diandric and digynic triploid genotypes on early mouse embryogenesis. Development 105:137–145, 1989.

6. Jacobs PA, Szulman AE, Funkhouser J, Matsuura JS, Wilson CC. Human triploidy: relationship between parental origin of the additional haploid complement and development of partial hydatiform mole. Ann Hum Genet 46:223–231, 1982.

7. Norris ML, Barton SC, Surani MA. The differential roles of parental genomes in mammalian development. Ox Rev Reprod Biol 12:225–244, 1990.

8. Solter D. Differential imprinting and expression of maternal and paternal genomes. Annu Rev Genet 22:127–146, 1988.

9. Thomson JA, Solter D. The developmental fate of androgenetic, parthenogenetic, and gynogenetic cells in chimeric gastrulating mouse embryos. Genes Dev 2:1344–1351, 1988.

10. McGrath J, Solter D. Completion of mouse embryogenesis requires both the maternal and paternal genomes. Cell 37:179–183, 1984.

11. Surani MA, Barton SC, Norris ML. Development of reconstituted mouse eggs suggests imprinting of the genome during gametogenesis. Nature 308:548–550, 1984.

12. Barton SC, Surani MAH, Norris ML. Role of paternal and maternal genomes in mouse development. Nature 311:374–376, 1984.

13. Lawler SD. Genetic studies on hydatidiform moles. Adv Exp Med Biol 176:147–161, 1984.

14. Kaufman MH, Speirs S, Lee KK. The sex-chromosome constitution and early postimplantation development of diandric triploid mouse embryos. Cytogenet Cell Genet 50:98–101, 1989.

15. McFadden DE, Kalousek DK. Two different phenotypes of fetuses with chromosomal triploidy: correlation with parental origin of the extra haploid set. Am J Med Genet 38:535–538, 1991.

16. Surani MA, Barton SC. Development of gynogenetic eggs in the mouse: implications for parthenogenetic embryos. Science 222:1034–1036, 1983.

17. Cattanach BM, Kirk M. Differential activity of maternally and paternally derived chromosome regions in mice. Nature 315:496–498, 1985.

18. Cattanach BM. Parental origin effects in mice. J Embryol Exp Morph 97 (Suppl):137–150, 1986.

19. Searle AG, Peters J, Lyon MF, Hall JG, Evans EP, Edwards JH, et al. Chromosome maps of man and mouse. IV. Ann Hum Genet 53:89–140, 1989.

20. McGrath J, Solter D. Maternal Thp lethality in the mouse is a nuclear, not cytoplasmic, defect. Nature 308:550–551, 1984.

21. Barlow DP, Stoger R, Herrmann BG, Saito K, Schweifer N. The mouse insulin-like growth factor type-2 receptor is imprinted and closely linked to the Tme locus. Nature 349:84–87, 1991.

22. MacDonald RG, Pfeffer SR, Coussens L, Tepper MA, Brocklebank CM, Mole JE, et al. A single receptor binds both insulin-like growth factor II and mannose-6-phosphate. Science 239:1134–1137, 1988.

23. Tong PY, Tollefsen SE, Kornfeld S. The cation-dependent mannose 6-phosphate receptor binds insulin-like growth factor II. J Biol Chem 263:2585–2588, 1988.

24. DeChiara TM, Robertson EJ, Efstratiadis A. Parental imprinting of the mouse insulin-like growth factor II gene. Cell 64:849–859, 1991.

25. DeChiara TM, Efstratiadis A, Robertson EJ. A growth-deficiency phenotype in heterozygous mice carrying an insulin-like growth factor II gene disrupted by targeting. Nature 345:78–80, 1990.

26. Bartolomei MS, Zemel S, Tilghman SM. Parental imprinting of the mouse H19 gene. Nature 351:153–155, 1991.

27. Brannan CI, Dees EC, Ingram RS, Tilghman SM. The product of the H19 gene may function as an RNA. Mol Cell Biol 10:28–36, 1990.

28. Brunkow ME, Tilghman SM. Ectopic expression of the H19 gene in mice causes prenatal lethality. Genes Dev 5:1092–1101, 1991.

29. Zemel S, Bartolomei MS, Tilghman SM. Physical linkage of two mammalian imprinted genes, H19 and insulin-like growth factor 2. Nat Genet 2:61–65, 1992.

30. Zhang Y, Tycko B. Monoallelic expression of the human H19 gene. Nat Genet 1:40–44, 1992.

31. Ohlsson R, Nystrom A, Pfeifer-Ohlsson S, Tohonen V, Hedborg F, Schofield P, et al. IGF2 is parentally imprinted during human embryogenesis and in the Beckwith-Wiedmann syndrome. Nat Genet 4:94–97, 1993.

32. Ferguson-Smith AC, Sasaki H, Cattanach BM, Surani MA. Parental-origin-specific epigenetic modification of the mouse H19 gene. Nature 362:751–755, 1993.

33. Chung W-Y, Yuan L, Feng L, Hensle T, Tycko B. Chromosome 11p15.5 regional imprinting: comparative analysis of KIP2 and H19 in human tissues and Wilms tumor. Hum Mol Genet 5:1101–1108, 1996.

34. Leighton PA, Saam JR, Ingram RS, Tilghman SM. Genomic imprinting in mice: its function and mechanism. Biol Reprod 54:273–278, 1996.

35. Ozcelik T, Leff S, Robinson W, Donlon T, Lalande M, Sanjines E. Small nuclear ribonuclear protein N (SNRPN), an expressed gene in the Prader-Willi syndrome critical region. Nat Genet 2:265–269, 1992.

36. Leff SE, Brannan CI, Reed ML, Ozcelik T, Francke U, Copeland NG. Maternal imprinting of the mouse Snrpn gene and conserved linkage homology with the human Prader-Willi syndrome region. Nat Genet 2:259–264, 1992.

37. Wevrick R, Kerns JA, Francke U. Identification of a novel paternally expressed gene in the Prader-Willi syndrome region. Hum Mol Genet 3:1877–1882, 1994.

38. Glenn CC, Nicholls RD, Robinson WP, Saitoh S, Niikawa N, Schinzel A, et al. Modification of 15q11-q13 DNA methylation imprints in unique Angelman and Prader-Willi patients. Hum Mol Genet 2:1377–1382, 1993.

39. Sutcliffe JS, Nakao M, Christian S, Orstavik KH, Tommerup N, Ledbetter DH, et al. Deletions of a differentially methylated CpG island at the SNRPN gene define a putative imprinting control region. Nat Genet 8:52–58, 1994.

40. Butler MG. Prader-Willi syndrome: current understanding of cause and diagnosis. Am J Med Genet 35:319–332, 1990.

41. Williams CA, Frias JL. The Angelman ("happy puppet") syndrome. Am J Med Genet 11:453–460, 1982.

42. Ledbetter DH, Riccardi VM, Airhard SD, Strobel RJ, Keenan BS, Crawford JD. Deletion of chromosome 15 as a cause of the Prader-Willi syndrome. N Engl J Med 304:325–329, 1981.

43. Driscoll DJ. Genomic imprinting in humans. Molec Genet Med 4:37–77, 1994.

44. Butler MG, Meany FJ, Palmer CG. Clinical and cytogenetic survey of 39 individuals with Prader-Labhart-Willi syndrome. Am J Med Genet 23:793–809, 1986.

45. Donlon TA. Similar molecular deletions on chromosome 15q11.2 are encountered in both the Prader-Willi and Angelman syndromes. Hum Genet 80:322–328, 1988.

46. Knoll JHM, Nicholls RD, Magenis RE, Graham JMJ, Lalande M, Latt SA. Angelman and Prader-Willi syndromes share a common chromosome 15 deletion but differ in parental origin of the deletion. Am J Med Genet 32:285–290, 1989.

47. Pembrey M, Fennell SJ, van-den-Berghe J, Fitchett M, Summers D, Butler L, et al.

The association of Angelman's syndrome with deletions within 15q11–13. J Med Genet 26:73–77, 1989.

48. Magenis RE, Toth-Fejel S, Allen LJ, Black M, Brown MG, Budden S, et al. Comparison of the 15q deletions in Prader-Willi and Angelman syndromes: specific regions, extent of deletions, parental origin, and clinical consequences. Am J Med Genet 35:333–349, 1990.

49. Williams CA, Zori RT, Stone JW, Gray BA, Cantu ES, Ostrer H. Maternal origin of 15q11–13 deletions in Angelman syndrome suggests a role for genomic imprinting. Am J Med Genet 35:350–353, 1990.

50. Nicholls RD, Knoll JH, Butler MG, Karam S, Lalande M. Genetic imprinting suggested by maternal heterodisomy in nondeletion Prader-Willi syndrome. Nature 342:281–285, 1989.

51. Robinson WP, Bottani A, Xie YG, Balakrishman J, Binkert F, Mächler M, et al. Molecular, cytogenetic, and clinical investigations of Prader-Willi syndrome patients. Am J Hum Genet 49:1219–1234, 1991.

52. Malcolm S, Clayton-Smith J, Nichols M, Robb S, Webb T, Armour JA, et al. Uniparental paternal disomy in Angelman's syndrome. Lancet 337:694–697, 1991.

53. Knoll JH, Glatt KA, Nicholls RD, Malcolm S, Lalande M. Chromosome 15 uniparental disomy is not frequent in Angelman syndrome. Am J Hum Genet 48:16–21, 1991.

54. Gregory CA, Schwartz J, Kirkilionis AJ, Rudd N, Hamerton JL. Somatic recombination rather than uniparental disomy suggested as another mechanism by which genetic imprinting may play a role in the etiology of Prader-Willi syndrome. Hum Genet 88:42–48, 1991.

55. Hulten M, Armstrong S, Challinor P, Gould C, Hardy G, Leedham P, et al. Genomic imprinting in an Angelman and Prader-Willi translocation family. Lancet 338:638–639, 1991.

56. Buiting K, Neumann M, Ludecke HJ, Senger G, Claussen U, Antich J, et al. Microdissection of the Prader-Willi syndrome chromosome region and identification of potential gene sequences. Genomics 6:521–527, 1990.

57. Schulze A, Hansen C, Skakkebaek NE, Brondrum-Nielsen K, Ledbetter DH, Tommerup N. Exclusion of SNRPN as a major determinant of Prader-Willi syndrome by a translocation breakpoint. Nat Genet 12:452–454, 1996.

58. Hamabe J, Kuroki Y, Imaizumi K, Sugimoto T, Fukushima Y, Yamaguchi A, et al. DNA deletion and its parental origin in Angelman syndrome patients. Am J Med Genet 41:64–68, 1991.

59. Matsuura T, Sutcliffe JS, Fang P, Galgarrd RJ, Jiang YH, Benton CS, et al. De novo truncating mutations in E—AO ubiquitin-protein ligase gene (UBE3A) in Angelman syndrome. Nat Genet 15:74–77, 1997.

60. Kishino T, Lalande M, Wagstaff J. UBE3A/E6-AP mutations cause Angelman syndrome. Nat Genet 15:70–73, 1997.

61. Wagstaff J, Knoll JH, Glatt KA, Shugart YY, Sommer A, Lalande M. Maternal but not paternal transmission of 15q11–13-linked nondeletion Angelman syndrome leads to phenotypic expression. Nat Genet 1:291–294, 1992.

62. Beckwith J. Macroglossia, omphalocele, adrenal cytomegaly, gigantism, and hyperplastic visceromegaly. Birth Defects Orig Art Ser 5:188–196, 1969.

63. Wiedemann H-R. Das EMG Syndrome: Exomphalos, Makroglossie, Gigantismus, und Kohlenhydratstoffwechselstoerung. Z Kinderheilk 106:171–185, 1969.

64. Kosseff AL, Hermann J, Gilbert EF, Visekul C, Lubinsky M, Opitz JM. Studies of malformation syndromes of man XXIX: the Wiedemann-Beckwith Syndrome. Clini-

cal, genetic and pathogenetic studies of 12 cases. Eur J Pediatr. 123:139–166, 1976.

65. Waiziri M, Patil SR, Hanson JW, Bartley JA. Abnormality of chromosome 11 in person with features of Beckwith-Wiedemann syndrome. J Pediatr 102:873–876, 1983.

66. Brown KW, Gardner A, Williams JC, Mott MG, McDermott A, Maitland NJ. Paternal origin of 11p15 duplications in the Beckwith-Wiedemann syndrome. A new case and review of the literature. Cancer Genet Cytogenet 58:66–70, 1992.

67. Henry I, Bonaiti Pellie C, Chehensse V, Beldjord C, Schwartz C, Utermann G, et al. Uniparental paternal disomy in a genetic cancer-predisposing syndrome. Nature 351:665–667, 1991.

68. Grundy P, Telzerow P, Paterson MC, Haber D, Berman B, Li F, et al. Chromosome 11 uniparental isodisomy predisposing to embryonal neoplasms. Lancet 338:1079–1080, 1991.

69. Nystrom A, Cheetham JE, Engstrom W, Schofield PN. Molecular analysis of patients with Wiedemann-Beckwith syndrome. II. Paternally derived disomies of chromosome 11. Eur J Pediatr 151:511–514, 1992.

70. Brown KW, Williams JC, Maitland NJ, Mott MG. Genomic imprinting and the Beckwith-Wiedemann syndrome. Am J Hum Genet 46:1000–1001, 1990.

71. Ping AJ, Reeve AE, Law DJ, Young MR, Boehnke M, Feinberg AP. Genetic linkage of Beckwith-Wiedemann syndrome to 11p15. Am J Hum Genet 44:720–723, 1989.

72. Koufos A, Grundy P, Morgan K, Aleck KA, Hadro T, Lampkin BC, et al. Familial Wiedemann-Beckwith syndrome and a second Wilms tumor locus both map to 11p15.5. Am J Hum Genet 44:711–719, 1989.

73. Aleck KA, Hadro TA. Dominant inheritance of Wiedemann-Beckwith Syndrome: further evidence for transmission of "unstable premutation" through carrier women. Am J Med Genet 33:155–160, 1989.

74. Weksberg R, Shen DR, Fei YL, Song QL, Squire J. Disruption of insulin-like growth factor 2 imprinting in Beckwith-Wiedmann syndrome. Nat Genet 5:143–150, 1993.

75. Ferguson-Smith AC, Cattanach BM, Barton SC, Beechey CV, Surani MA. Embryological and molecular investigations of parental imprinting on mouse chromosome 7. Nature 351:667–670, 1991.

76. Riccardi VM, Sujansky E, Smith AC, Francke U. Chromosomal imbalance in the Aniridia-Wilms' tumor association: 11p interstitial deletion. Pediatrics 61:604–610, 1978.

77. Schroeder WT, Chao LY, Dao DD, Strong LC, Pathak S, Riccardi V, et al. Nonrandom loss of maternal chromosome 11 alleles in Wilms tumors. Am J Hum Genet 40:413–420, 1987.

78. Huff V, Meadows A, Riccardi VM, Strong LC, Saunders GF. Parental origin of de novo constitutional deletions of chromosomal band 11p13. Am J Hum Genet 47:155–160, 1990.

79. Wilkins RJ. Genomic imprinting and carcinogenesis. Lancet 1:329–331, 1988.

80. Mannens M, Slater RM, Heyting C, Bliek J, de Kraker J, Coad N, et al. Molecular nature of genetic changes resulting in loss of heterozygosity of chromosome 11 in Wilms' tumour. Hum Genet 81:41–48, 1988.

81. Scrable HJ, Witte DP, Lampkin BC, Cavenee WK. Chromosomal localization of the human rhabdomyosarcoma locus by mitotic recombination mapping. Nature 329:645–647, 1987.

82. Scrable H, Cavenee W, Ghavimi F, Lovell M, Morgan K, Sapienza C. A model for

embryonal rhabdomyosarcoma tumorigenesis that involves genome imprinting. Proc Natl Acad Sci USA Oct; 86(19):7480–7484, 1989.

83. Gerschensen LE, Rotello RJ. Apoptosis: a different type of cell death. FASEB J 6:2450–2455, 1992.

84. Rainier S, Johnson LA, Dobry CJ, Ping AJ, Grundy PE, Feinberg AP. Relaxation of imprinted genes in human cancer. Nature 362:747–749, 1993.

85. Zhang Y, Shields T, Crenshaw T, Hao Y, Moulton T, Tycko B. Imprinting of human H19: Allele-specific CpG methylation, loss of active allele in Wilms tumor, and potential for somatic allele switching. Am J Hum Genet 53:113–124, 1995.

86. Ogawa O, Eccles MR, Szeto J, McNoe LA, Yun K, Maw MA, et al. Relaxation of insulin-like growth factor II gene imprinting implicated in Wilms' tumor. Nature 362:749–751, 1993.

87. Moulton T, Crenshaw T, Hao Y, Moosikasuwan J, Lin N, Dembitzer F. Epigenetic lesions at the H19 locus in Wilms' tumor patients. Nat Genet 7:440–447, 1994.

88. Steenman MJC, Rainier S, Dobry CJ, Grundy P, Horon IL, Feinberg AP. Loss of imprinting of IGF2 is linked to reduced expression and abnormal methylation of H19 in Wilms' tumor. Nat Genet 7:433–439, 1994.

89. Taniguchi T, Sullivan MJ, Osamu O, Reeve A. Epigenetic changes encompassing the IGF2/H19 locus associated with relaxation of the IGF2 imprinting and silencing of H19 in Wilms tumor. Proc Natl Acad Sci USA 92:2159–2163, 1995.

90. Hao Y, Crenshaw T, Moulton T, Newcomb E, Tycko B. Tumor suppressor activity of H19 RNA. Nature 365:764–767, 1993.

91. van der Mey AG, Maaswinkel-Mooy PD, Cornelisse CJ, Schmidt PH, van de Kamp JJ. Genomic imprinting in hereditary glomus tumours: evidence for new genetic theory. Lancet 2:1291–1294, 1989.

92. Heutink P, van der Mey AGL, Sandkuijl A, van Gils APG, Bardoel A, Breedveld GJ. A gene subject to genomic imprinting and responsible for hereditary paragangliomas maps to chromosome 11q23-qter. Hum Mol Genet 1:7–10, 1992.

93. Bird AP. CpG-rich islands and the function of DNA methylation. Nature 321:209–213, 1986.

94. Driscoll DJ, Migeon BR. Sex difference in methylation of single-copy genes in human meiotic germ cells: implication for X chromosome inactivation, parental imprinting, and origin of CpG mutations. Somat Cell Mol Genet 16 (3):267–282, 1990.

95. Riggs AD. X inactivation, differentiation and DNA methylation. Cytogenet Cell Genet 14:9–25, 1975.

96. Pfeifer GP, Steigerwald SD, Mueller PR, Wold B, Riggs AD. Genomic sequencing and methylation analysis by ligation mediated PCR. Science 246:810–813, 1989.

97. Sapienza C, Peterson AC, Rossant J, Balling R. Degree of methylation of transgenes is dependent on gamete of origin. Nature 328:251–254, 1987.

98. Reik W, Collick A, Norris ML, Barton SC, Surani MA. Genomic imprinting determines methylation of parental alleles in transgenic mice. Nature 328:248–251, 1987.

99. Sapienza C, Paquette J, Tran TH, Peterson A. Epigenetic and genetic factors affect transgene methylation imprinting. Development 107:165–168, 1989.

100. Swain JL, Stewart TA, Leder P. Parental legacy determines methylation and expression of an autosomal transgene: a molecular mechanism for parental imprinting. Cell 50:719–727, 1987.

101. Chaillet JR, Vogt TF, Beier DR, Leder P. Parental-specific methylation of an im-

printed transgene is established during gametogenesis and progressively changes during embryogenesis. Cell 66:77–83, 1991.

102. Hadchouel M, Farza H, Simon D, Tiollias P, Pourcel C. Maternal inhibiotion of hepatitis B surface antigen gene expression in transgenic mice correlates with de novo methylation. Nature 329:454–456, 1987.

103. Sasaki H, Jones PA, Chaillet JR, Ferguson-Smith AC, Barton SC, Reik W, et al. Parental imprinting: potentially active chromatin of the repressed maternal allele of the mouse insulin-like growth factor II (Igf2) gene. Genes Dev 6:1843–1856, 1992.

104. Stoger R, Kubicka P, Liu C-G, Kafri T, Razin A, Cedar H, et al. Maternal-specific methylation of the imprinted mouse Igf2r locus identifies the expressed locus as carrying the imprinting signal. Cell 73:61–71, 1993.

105. Li E, Bestor TH, Jaenisch R. Targeted mutation of the DNA methyltransferase gene results in embryonic lethality. Cell 69:915–926, 1992.

106. Selig S, Okumura K, Ward DC, Cedar H. Delineation of DNA replication time zones by fluorescence in situ hybridization. EMBO J 11:1217–1225, 1992.

107. Kitsberg D, Selig S, Brandeis M, Simon I, Keshet I, Driscoll DJ, et al. Allele-specific replication timing of imprinted gene regions. Nature 364:459–463, 1993.

108. Sapienza C. Sex-linked dosage-sensitive modifiers as imprinting genes. Development Suppl:107–113, 1990.

109. Sapienza C. Genome imprinting, cellular mosaicism and carcinogenesis. Mol Carcinog 3:118–121, 1990.

110. Klar AJ. Regulation of fission yeast mating-type interconversion by chromosome imprinting. Development—(Suppl): 3–8, 1990.

8

Accelerated Rates of Mutation

The rate of mutation may be accelerated so that new alleles form in a high proportion of daughter cells. An increased rate of mutation may be a feature of a gene's structure, which causes its replication to be unfaithful. These structures are commonly referred to as *premutations.*[1,2] Alternatively, the machinery for replicating DNA or for repairing replication errors may be flawed as the result of a cell's genetic constitution or its exposure to mutagenic agents. When these processes alter a mutant gene in the germ line, some offspring are nonpenetrant, whereas others are more severely affected than their parents. If the alteration of a gene occurs preferentially in either an egg or a sperm cell, then there may be a parent-of-origin effect. When these defects occur in gametes or in embryonic somatic cells, they may cause developmental abnormalities. When the mutations occur in somatic cells, they may be lethal to the cell, or they may confer a growth advantage and may even cause the cell to be malignant.

DYNAMIC MUTATION IN GERM CELLS

Transmission of unstable premutations. Transmission of unstable premutations that progress to full mutations was postulated to account for unaffected or mildly affected progenitors having severely affected descendants. Among the diseases for which this occurrs are myotonic dystrophy and fragile X syndrome.

Anticipation. The phenomenon in which a genetic condition appears to worsen in subsequent generations is known as *anticipation.*[3] The concept of anticipation existed from the beginning of human genetics as a discipline. As Penrose noted, "The idea has had considerable backing in traditions and according to Galton (1869) could even apply to good qualities wherein sons were more precocious than their gifted fathers."[4] During the early part of the 20th-century, the concept was extended by eugenicists to explain their concept of degeneration of the germ plasm as the basis for familial mental retardation and mental illness. For example, Mott observed that "more than one-half of the insane offspring of insane parents are congenital idiots or imbeciles."[3] Because eugenicists employed nonrigorous methods, the validity of the concept was challenged.[4]

From the earliest clinical description, myotonic dystrophy (DM) was suspected of showing anticipation.[4-8] Myotonic dystrophy is an autosomal dominant condition that is characterized by uncontrollable contraction of the muscles and progressive muscle weakness and wasting especially in the temporal and neck muscles. Affected individuals may also have cataracts, hypogonadism, frontal balding, mental retardation, and heart block. In 1918, Bernhardt Fleischer laid out the criteria for anticipation in myotonic dystrophy. He suggested that cataract in later life was the major feature in the first affected generation and that muscle disease might occur in subsequent generations.[9]

In the 1940s Julia Bell demonstrated anticipation in myotonic dystrophy.[6] She discerned a stronger correlation for the age of onset of disease between affected siblings than between affected parent and sibling pairs. She also demonstrated that the age of onset was earlier in the second generation than in the first. Despite her use of quantitative methods, her conclusions were disputed by Penrose, who suggested that the data could be explained by ascertainment biases.[4] These were identification of parents with late-onset disease (early onset of disease would diminish fertility), identification of children with early onset

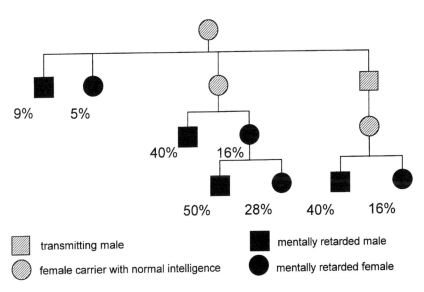

Figure 8.1. Transmission of the fragile X syndrome demonstrating the Sherman paradox. The percentages indicate the likelihood of a mentally retarded offspring.

disease, and identification of parents and children with simultaneous onset. Although never observed, he postulated the existence of families with early onset disease in parents and late-onset disease in children.

The most severe case of anticipation in DM is congenital or early onset disease (age less than 5 years). These children have severe hypotonia, facial weakness and mental retardation, and usually die at less than a year of age from respiratory failure.[8] The transmission of early onset DM is affected by parental origin. In 34 of 35 cases, Harper and Dyken demonstrated that the affected parent was the mother. They postulated that the affected mothers might transmit a factor across the placenta that would influence the expression of the myotonic dystrophy gene or would have secondary adverse consequences on the fetus.[10]

The risk that any heterozygous woman with DM will have a child with congenital disease is 3–9%. The major factor determining the outcome in the infant is the clinical status of the mother at the time of pregnancy and delivery. Only women with multisystem disease have congenitally affected children. Heterozygous women with polychromatic lens changes as the only features of disease do not have congenitally affected children. Women with systemic disease are at 41% risk for having a congenitally affected child.[11]

Fragile X is the most common Mendelian cause of mental retardation and the second most common genetic cause of mental retardation after Down syndrome.[2] This X-linked condition affects approximately one in 2,000 males. The features of fragile X syndrome include moderate-to-severe mental retardation, prognathism, large ears, and macroorchidism.[12] A marker for the condition is the expression of a fragile site on the X chromosome at band Xq27.[13] The severity of mental retardation in affected individuals tends to worsen in later generations.[14,15] Females as well as males have mental retardation, despite random inactivation of the X chromosome.

Fragile X syndrome also demonstrates anticipation in a phenomenon that is known as the "Sherman paradox" (Fig. 8.1).[14,15] New fragile X mutations do not occur in affected males. Rather, all appear to be inherited from carrier females. The sons of female carriers have a 50% risk of inheriting the gene for the condition but only a 40% risk of being mentally retarded. The males who inherit the fragile X mutation, but are not mentally retarded, are known as "transmitting" males. Among females who inherit the fragile X mutation, approximately 35% are mentally retarded. If the heterozygous mother is mentally retarded, the likelihood of mental retardation in the daughter is increased from 16 to 28%. The phenotypes of the parents influence the phenotypes of the offspring. The likelihood that the daughter of a transmitting male is mentally retarded is less than 1%. If the heterozygous mother is mentally retarded the likelihood of mental retardation in the son is increased from 9 to 50%.

For both males and females, the likelihood of mental retardation correlates with their position in the pedigree. Transmitting males tend to be clustered in the earlier generations of the pedigrees and mentally retarded males in later generations. The children of the mothers of transmitting males have a lower risk of mental retardation than the children of daughters of transmitting males.

In 1985, Pembrey, Winter, and Davies developed a model to explain how an unstable premutation leads to the development of a full mutation that is associated with the mental retardation and other phenotypic features of fragile X syndrome.[1] They postulated that a premutation exists in an unaffected carrier male which becomes a full mutation only when transmitted in the germ cells of his daughters. They suggested that this premutation consists of a submicroscopic rearrangement at the fragile site on the distal long arm of the X chromosome that causes no ill effects per se but generates a significant imbalance when involved in a recombinational event with the other X chromosome. Nussbaum, Airhart, and Ledbetter suggested that the site for the premutation involves a pyrimidine-rich sequence present on normal X chromosomes.[16] Through the mechanism of nonhomologous recombination, this pyrimidine-rich sequence is amplified to produce the premutation in fragile X syndrome. Further amplification resulting in an even longer stretch of pyrimidine-rich sequence results in the full mutation.

Molecular mechanism of premutation and progression to full mutation. Amplification of a CG-rich sequence has been shown to be the mechanism of premutation and progression to full mutation in fragile X syndrome.[17-19] The polymorphic triplet repeat, CGG, is located upstream to the initiation codon of the FMR-1 gene (Fig. 8.2). From six to 54 copies of this CGG repeat have been found in the normal population. Individuals with the premutation, transmitting males and their carrier daughters, have 52–200 copies of the repeat. When transmitted to offspring, two types of instability have been identified in

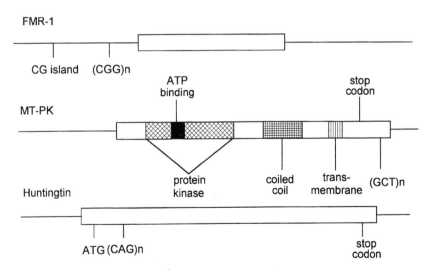

Figure 8.2. Structure of the FMR-1, MT-PK, and Huntington disease genes showing the location of the trinucleotide repeats.

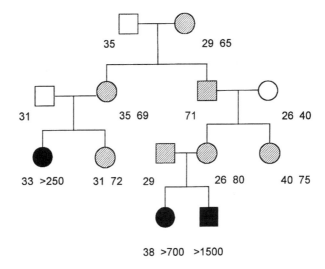

38 >700 >1500

☐ ◯ Normal

▨ ◍ Unaffected carrier

■ ● Mentally retarded individual

Figure 8.3. Transmission and amplification of the premutation in fragile X syndrome. The numbers indicate the copy numbers of the trinucleotide repeats.

the CGG repeat in the FMR-1 gene (Fig. 8.3). When transmitted from father to daughter, the size of this premutation may increase or decrease slightly. When transmitted from females with the premutation to their male or female progeny, the copy number may increase either slightly or dramatically to hundreds or even thousands of copies. This high copy number repeat is the full mutation in males and females with mental retardation.

Several factors influence the progression from premutation to full mutation. The first is maternal transmission. The second is the length of the CGG repeat in the premutation (Fig. 8.4).[20] CGG repeats that are interrupted by the AGG trinucleotide are less likely to undergo expansion to full mutation. The major determinant is the length of the CGG repeat on the 3' side of the interruption.[21] In addition, the FMR-1 gene is in linkage disequilibrium with polymorphic flanking markers. These alleles may be indicative of whether the repeat is interrupted.[22,23] Alternatively, they may be indicative of other regions of the X chromosome that influence expansion of the premutation.

Although it has been assumed that progression from the premutation to the full mutation may occur in oocytes, this need not be the case. Four males with fragile X syndrome had only premutation alleles in their sperm.[24] This can be explained by reversion of full-mutation alleles or by expansion from premuta-

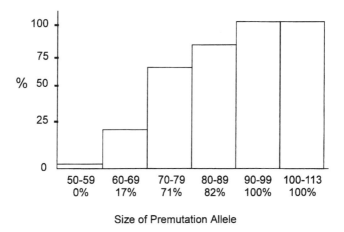

Figure 8.4. Fragile X syndrome: Likelihood of expansion to full mutation based on size of premutation.[17]

tion to full mutation that occurred in the zygote or early embryonic somatic cells. If this is the case, these individuals inherited an FMR-1 gene from their mothers that was marked with a tendency toward expansion.

Expansion of a trinucleotide repeat (GCT) is also the mechanism of mutation in myotonic dystrophy.[25–28] In the normal population, the size of the repeat is five to 27 copies (Fig. 8.5). Individuals with 50–100 copies of the repeat have mild or no symptoms. Individuals with greater than 100 copies to several thousand copies have systemic manifestations of myotonic dystrophy.[25,26,28] Children with congenital myotonic dystrophy have CTG repeats that are longer on average than those found in individuals with later onset disease.[29] Expansion of the trinucleotide repeat occurs in the germ cells of males and females. The size of the parental alleles correlates with the likelihood of expansion. The alleles that are transmitted by males tend to be longer than those transmitted by females, although very long alleles are selected again via spermatocytes.[30] Other regions of the genome in the vicinity of the myotonic dystrophy locus may influence the expansion because strong linkage disequilibrium has been observed with nearby markers.[31,32] Very long alleles are not transmitted by affected males who are infertile.

On the basis of this work, expansion of trinucleotide repeats has become a hallmark for identifying genes for other conditions that demonstrate anticipation, including Huntington disease, spinocerebellar ataxia types I and II, dentatorubral and pallidoluysian atrophy, and Marchado-Joseph disease.[33–39] Huntington disease is a progressive neurodegenerative disorder that is characterized by choreiform movements, cognitive dysfunction, and emotional disturbance.[40] The more severe juvenile form occurs prior to the age of 21 and is characterized by the development of rigidity. This form of the disease is transmitted almost always by an affected father.[41,42] The gene for Huntington disease

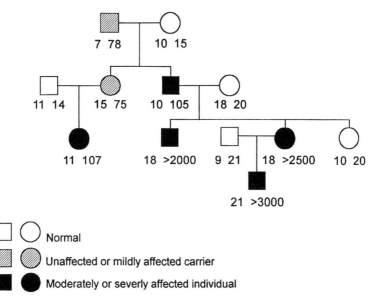

Figure 8.5. Transmission and amplification of the premutation in myotonic dystrophy. The numbers indicate the copy numbers of the trinucleotide repeats.

contains a CAG trinucleotide repeat at the 3' end, encoding a C-terminal polyglutamine track.[43] Normal individuals tend to have trinucleotide repeat copy numbers of 37 or less, whereas affected individuals have copy numbers of 42 or more. The length of the repeat correlates with the age of onset of the disease.[44] Juvenile-onset disease is characterized by 100 or more copies, generally the greatest copy numbers that are observed among individuals with HD. Paternally transmitted alleles are more likely to expand and therefore tend to be longer.

The features of spinocerebellar atrophy I include ataxia, ophthalmoparesis, and variable motor weakness.[45] The disease results from degeneration of the neurons in the cerebellar cortex, dentate nuclei, and brainstem. The mechanism of mutation is expansion of a CAG repeat that is present at the 3' coding region of a gene on the short arm of chromosome 6, termed *ataxin-1*.[34,35] Normal alleles have 19–36 copies of the repeat, whereas SCA1 alleles have 43–81 copies. The age of onset correlates inversely with the length of the trinucleotide repeat. Paternally transmitted alleles are more likely to expand than maternally transmitted alleles. Alleles in which the trinucleotide repeat is interrupted are less likely to expand.

Dentatorubral-pallidoluysian atrophy (DRPLA) is a condition that occurs predominantly among Japanese individuals and presents with myoclonic epilepsy, dementia, ataxia, and choreoathetosis. The symptoms result from degeneration of the dentate nucleus, microcalcification of the globus pallidus, demyelination of the centrum semiovale, and neuronal dystrophy of the posterior columns.[46] The disorder results from expansion of a CAG trinucleotide repeat in a gene of unknown function that maps to chromosome 12.[37,38] Normal individuals have seven to 23 copies of the repeat whereas affected individuals have 49–75 copies, or occasionally even more. The age of onset is earlier and the severity of the symptoms is worse in individuals who have greater numbers of repeats.

Expansion of trinucleotide repeats has also been observed in X-linked spinal and bulbar muscular atrophy (SBMA) and in fragile X E mental retardation (FRAXE), although anticipation has not been demonstrated for these disorders.[47,48] SBMA is an adult-onset motor neuron disease that is characterized by progressive weakness in the upper and lower extremities.[49] Affected individuals have proximal muscle weakness, intention tremor, muscle cramps, and dysphagia. A triplet repeat, CAG is found in exon 1 of the androgen receptor gene. In the normal population there are 17–26 copies of this repeat, whereas in the males affected with SBMA the copy number is 40–52.[47] There is greater instability with paternal than with maternal transmission. The size of allele correlates with the likelihood of expansion, although, in sperm, contractions are more likely than expansions.

Individuals with FRAXE syndrome have mild mental retardation and the characteristic fragile site on the distal long arm of the X chromosome that is induced in low folate medium; however, these individuals lack mutations in their FMR-1 gene.[50] The mental retardation in these individuals and their family members is on the basis of expansion of a CGG trinucleotide repeat in a gene that is 150–600 kb distal to the FMR-1 gene.[48] Normal individuals have six to 25 copies of the repeat whereas affected persons have greater than 200 copies. The length of the repeat usually decreases when passed from a male to a carrier daughter and increases when passed from a female to an affected son.

Expansion of trinucleotide repeats is likely to be found as the mechanism of mutation in other human diseases. More than 12 gene sequences in GenBank have copies of the CCA and AAT repeats.[51,52] The use of trinucleotide repeats as hybridization probes has revealed more than 40 independent cDNA clones in human libraries. For conditions for which expansion of trinucleotide repeats is suspected to be the mechanism of mutation, candidate genes that map to the same region of the genome as the disease locus can be tested by linkage of the expansion to the disease phenotype.

Trinucleotide repeats and disease pathogenesis. The role of expansion of the trinucleotide repeat in the pathogenesis of these various conditions is not likely to be the same because the expansion occurs in different regions of the respective genes. For some diseases, the effect may be decreased expression of the candidate gene, whereas for others novel protein products may be produced.

The FMR-1 gene encodes a cytosolic RNA-binding protein. The gene is transcribed in brain and in other tissues. Expansion of the trinucleotide repeat results in decreased transcription of the FMR-1 mRNA. The expansion of the trinucleotide repeat correlates with the decrease in transcription and with methylation of a CG island 200 bp upstream from the transcription initiation site of the FMR-1 gene; hence, the FMR-1 gene appears to be displaced from its 5' regulatory region, which contains CG dinucleotides that are methylated and in the inactive state (Fig. 8.2).

For a number of these disorders, expansion of a trinucleotide repeat results in an increase in the number of residues of a given amino acid. In Huntington disease, SCA1, DRPLA, and SBMA, the expansion of the CAG trinucleotide repeat results in a lengthened polyglutamine track (Fig. 8.2).[35,37,38,43,47] Glutamine-rich regions are found in certain transcription factors, including Sp1, fushi tarazu, and the mouse Sry gene.[53,54] Some of these transcription factors act by binding to the TATA-binding protein, or other transcription factors, resulting in the formation of a transcription complex; hence, one effect of expansion of the glutamine repeat may cause the products encoded by the genes to become transcription factors. Alternatively, through their interactions with transcription factors, these proteins may sequester or inhibit transcription factors that normally play a physiologic role.

The role of the MT-PK gene in the development of myotonic dystrophy is unknown. Based on homology with other sequences, the MT-PK gene encodes a protein that has an ATP-binding site, a catalytic domain for a protein kinase, and a transmembrane region (Fig. 8.2). The gene is highly expressed in skeletal and cardiac muscle, where it may act as a signal transduction protein. The expansion of the trinucleotide repeat in the MT-PK gene occurs in the 3' noncoding region of the mRNA. The presence of this repeat may decrease the stability of the mRNA.

Mechanisms of expansion for trinucleotide repeats. Several different mechanisms have been proposed for expansion of trinucleotide repeats. One is replication slippage. This occurs when the RNA fragment that primes DNA synthesis slips forward or back by one or more repeat lengths during replication. The result is a small gain or loss in the number of repeats. Because recombination is not involved, there is no alteration in the phase of the flanking markers. An alternative, but similar, mechanism is "breathing" of the newly synthesized DNA fragment. The newly synthesized fragment may separate from the parent strand, then reanneal the trinucleotide repeat at different sites, resulting in single-stranded bubbles in the parent and daughter strands. Through both mechanisms, the length of the new alleles would vary from the parental allele by a multiple of 3 bp. Longer alleles would be more likely to undergo slippage and form stable heteroduplexes. Alleles that have interrupted trinucleotide repeats would form less stable heteroduplexes and therefore would be less likely to be propagated to offspring.

An alternative mechanism for generating the somatic variation is unequal recombination between the two homologous chromosomes of a given pair. If the two chromatids are misaligned, the effect of recombination is to generate one chromatid with a duplication and the other with a deficiency. The maximum increase in copy number is up to twofold. Repetition of the process may result in a large number of fragments of different sizes. If the observed increase in the rate of sister chromatid exchange in fragile X syndrome occurs at the CGG repeat, this may account for the wide variation in the sizes of the repeats that are observed in somatic cells.

The "onion skin" model involving multiple rounds of unscheduled DNA synthesis has been proposed to account for the progression from premutation to full mutation.[55] In this model multiple rounds of initiation occur at a site that is adjacent to the triplet repeat. This generates a set of replication bubbles. These replication intermediates are unstable and subsequently recombined to form a longer repeat unit. This can result in the large increases in copy number that are observed in full mutations. Because the sites of recombination may not occur faithfully at the end of the triplet repeat, there may be a shift in the repetition of the trinucleotide at the sites of recombination.

Linkage disequilibrium between disease alleles and alleles of linked markers suggests that sequences outside the trinucleotide repeat may determine which repeats are susceptible to amplification. [23,31,32] Alternatively, the linkage disequilibrium may reflect the population history of random mutations. In the case of myotonic dystrophy in the French-Canadian population, all of the affected individuals are thought to have descended from a single founder.[32]

ACCELERATED RATES OF MUTATION IN SOMATIC CELLS

Unstable structures. Errors in replication may occur at the somatic level as well as in germ cells. Some of the errors may be intrinsic to the structure of specific genes or to chromosomal structures. Dinucleotide and trinucleotide repeats have unstable structures in somatic cells. Through slips in replication, a host of alleles of different sizes may be generated. Although these new alleles may be assumed to affect the disease phenotype, this has not been observed for myotonic dystrophy. The progression of this disorder with age does not appear to correlate with defects in replication.[56]

Human telomeres are made up of random copies of the repeated sequence TTAGGG. These structures provide physical ends to chromosomes, thus preventing the attachment of noncontiguous chromosomal ends.[57] Telomeres have the property of folding back on themselves. With increasing age of the host, the replication of the telomeres is faulty, resulting in shortening of the repeats. The rate of loss is approximately 30 bp per year. Telomere length is the best-known molecular predictor of the residual capacity of human fibroblasts to replicate.[58]

The enzyme telomerase ordinarily adds multiple repeats to the end of a telomere by using an RNA template.[59] This enzyme is not expressed in most somatic cells. Telomerase activity is present in human cell lines that have unlimited growth potential. Some tumor cells including colorectal adenomas and carcinomas and breast carcinomas have shortened, but stable, telomeres and telomerase activity. It has been suggested that cancer cells lose telomeric DNA up to a critical point. In some cells in which telomerase gene expression is derepressed and enzyme activity is restored, selective replication occurs.[60]

Telomerase can heal the ends of broken chromosomes, thereby allowing for their stable inheritance. In one case of α-thalassemia with mental retardation, a loss of the terminal 2 Mb of the chromosome was associated with the addition of a telomere repeat, resulting in stable transmission of that chromosome and pure monosomy for the distal chromosome 16p.[61]

The correlation between telomere loss and replication decline for somatic cells may play a role in some of the diseases of aging. Acceleration in the rate of telomere reduction has been observed in the lymphocytes of individuals with Down syndrome, a condition that is associated with premature aging.[62] Although fibroblast-type cells are thought to have a lifespan of 50 population doublings, the variability within a population of cells or between different cell types can be quite large.[63] In some tissues, loss of replication of one cell type may be associated with overgrowth of other cell types with tissue replacement or scarring. As a result, loss of replication competence may play a role in age-related vascular disease, immunodeficiency, or degenerative disease, such as osteoarthritis.

Faulty repair. Certain genetic disorders occur as the result of defects in the proofreading or repair of errors in DNA synthesis during replication. These conditions have a *mutator phenotype* that is associated either with somatic abnormalities that are specific to the condition or with a higher frequency of cancers in the affected individuals or both (Fig. 8.6). Two different DNA repair pathways have been discerned. Mismatch repair corrects errors that occur while DNA is being copied, usually from insertion of the wrong nucleotide at a given site. Nucleotide excision repair removes and replaces thymine dimers that have formed while exposing dividing cells to UV light, ionizing radiation, or chemicals.

Hereditary nonpolyposis colorectal cancer (HNPCC) is a dominant condition in which heterozygotes for HNPCC have an increased risk for right-sided colon, breast, ovarian, and endometrial tumors.[64] The tumor DNA in these individuals has a high frequency of replication errors, which results in variation in the size of dinucleotide CA markers in the tumor compared to the germ line.[65] This instability in the microsatellite DNA of these tumors is a marker for a

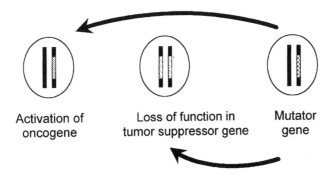

Activation of oncogene   Loss of function in tumor suppressor gene   Mutator gene

Figure 8.6. Mechanisms of tumor pathogenesis.

defect in mismatch repair. Based on this observation, defects in proteins that play a role in mismatched repair were identified.

Almost all cases of HNPCC arise from mutations in the MLH1 or MSH2 or PMS1 or PMS2 gene.[66-70] These genes have homologues in yeast and in *E. coli*, where they are known to play a role in the repair of mismatched nucleotides that occur as the result of deamination of 5-methylcytosine, misincorporation of bases during DNA synthesis, or mismatch between the heteroduplexes that form during genetic recombination (Fig. 8.7). Mutation in the yeast homologues of these genes results in an increased rate of expansion and contraction of dinucleotide repeated sequences. Further support for the idea that defects in mismatch repair play a role in the development of tumors in individuals with HNPCC has come from the observation that tumor cells with microsatellite instability are unable to carry out mismatch repair.[71]

Xeroderma pigmentosa (XP) is a condition of photosensitivity in which individuals develop rashes and subsequently tumors in the regions of sun-exposed skin.[73] This condition results from a defect in the nucleotide excision repair of thymidine dimers that form in response to exposure to UV light.[74] Ordinarily, these dimers require excision and repair for normal replication to proceed.[75] By fusing cultured somatic cells from affected individuals at least seven different complementation groups have been identified.[76] The XPA protein recognizes and binds to damaged DNA.[77] The XPB and XPD proteins are helicases that unwind the double-stranded DNA molecule.[78,79] XPF and a gene so far unre-

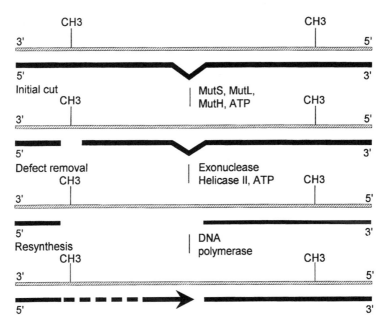

Figure 8.7. The pathway of mismatch repair of DNA.[71]

lated to xeroderma pigmentosa cut the 5' side of the damaged DNA.[80] XPG cuts the 3' side of the damaged DNA. A total stretch of 30 nucleotides is exercised, and then repaired using the cell's DNA synthetic enzymes.[81]

Other conditions have been associated with chromosomal instability in somatic cells. The basis for this assumption has been the occurrence of a higher frequency of chromosomal breaks and exchanges in the cultured cells of these individuals and the occurrence of a higher frequency of cancer. These conditions include Fanconi pancytopenia, Bloom syndrome, and ataxia telangiectasia.[82]

The defects in Fanconi pancytopenia include bone marrow failure, short stature, malformations of the heart, kidney and limbs (especially radii), and an increased risk of malignancy, especially acute myelogenous leukemia.[83] The spectrum of malformations can be highly variable and may be the result of somatic mutation and mosaicism.[84] Individuals with this condition have a defect in DNA repair which is manifested in two ways. First, the G2 phase of the cell cycle is very long.[85] Second, there is an increased frequency of chromosomal breaks when cells cultured from affected individuals are exposed to diepoxybutane.[86] The gene that cause two forms of Fanconi pancytopenia (complementation groups A and C) has been identified, although the role that they play in DNA repair has not been determined so far. [87,88]

The defects in Bloom syndrome include short stature and the development of rashes on sun-exposed skin surfaces.[89] Like Fanconi anemia, there is a predisposition to malignancy. Unlike Fanconi anemia, where the chromosomal breakage is seemingly random, the chromosomal aberrations in Bloom syndrome are between homologous chromosomes and are manifested as an increased frequency of sister chromatid exchanges (SCE).[82] In addition to high SCE lymphocytes, some people have a minor population of circulating low SCE cells. Analysis of genetic markers has demonstrated that these low SCE cells had a somatic recombination of chromosome 15 in a gene that has become known as *BLM*.[90] Somatic recombination between the sites of the maternally and paternally derived mutations results in the presence of a wild-type gene and the development of a low-SCE phenotype. The BLM gene has been shown to be homologous to RecQ helicases, a subfamily of DNA and RNA helicases. [91]

The defects in ataxia telangiectasia (AT) include telangiectasias in the sclerae and lungs of affected individuals, progressive ataxia, and rashes on sun-exposed areas. People with this condition are at increased risk for developing both acute and chromic lymphocytic leukemia.[92] Translocations of chromosome 14 involving band 14q32.1 are commonly observed in AT.[93] In addition, the G1-S checkpoint is abolished in the cells from patients with AT.[94] This checkpoint delays the progress of cells into S phase, thereby allowing repair of DNA damage, which would be perpetuated in the absence of the checkpoint. This checkpoint and the G2-M checkpoint are thought to consist of surveillance mechanisms for DNA damage, signal transduction pathways that amplify and transmit the signal to the replication or segregation machinery, and possibly repair activities. The delay in G2 in Fanconi anemia cells suggests that these cells may have a checkpoint defect, but unlike AT cells, it is at G2-M. Obligate heterozygous for AT have been observed to have an increased frequency of breast cancer.[95] Somatic mutation of the wild type AT gene in these heterozygotes would lead to a population of cells in which the G1-S checkpoint has been abolished. Thus, these cells may be more susceptible to transmitting somatic mutations.

Gene amplification. A common form of mutation in tumor cells is gene amplification. The inherent instability of the genomes of tumor cells favors progression from a less malignant to a more malignant phenotype. This process is seemingly a vicious cycle, because genomic instability seems to increase as tumor cells achieve a higher state of malignancy. This increase in genome instability is genetically controlled and may be a requirement for gene amplification to occur. Moreover, amplification of specific genes may contribute to the development of genome instability.

Amplification has been observed for members of three different classes of genes, including growth factors and their receptors, and drug resistance genes. Amplification of the erb-B2 oncogene, a truncated form of the epidermal growth factor receptor gene, has been observed in advance stages of breast and ovarian cancer.[94] Amplification of the N-myc growth factor gene occurs in later stages of neuroblastoma (stages 3 and 4).[97] For all of these conditions, gene amplification is a poor prognostic sign. The MDRI gene encodes a P-glycoprotein with broad specificity as an efflux pump. Amplification of this gene causes resistance to multiple drugs, including cancer chemotherapy agents.[98]

Amplification of a chromosomal region may involve more than one gene that affects the phenotype. The MDM-2 gene encodes a protein that specifically binds and inactivates the product of the p53 tumor suppressor gene.[99] In some human sarcomas, the region of gene amplification includes not only MDM2 but also the nearby CDK4 and GLI genes.[100] CDK4 is a cyclin-dependent kinase and is a major catalytic subunit whose activity enforces the commitment of cells to enter S phase.[101] The GLI gene encodes a zinc-finger DNA-binding protein, whose expression is developmentally regulated.[102]

Gene amplification appears to occur extrachromosomally. The amplified fragment may then reintegrate into a host chromosome, although not necessarily at the original site.[103] The extrachromosomal fragments are recognized as double minute chromosomes (dm) and reintegrants are recognized as homogeneously staining regions (HSR) of chromosomes.[104] Double minute chromosomes are small, independently replicating chromosomal structures whose copy number may vary from one cell to the next. Homogeneously staining regions (HSRs), as their name suggests, are nonbanding regions of chromosomes that are found in tumor cells, but not their parental cell type. Both HSRs and dms have been found to contain regions of DNA that have been amplified hundreds to thousands of times. Double minute chromosomes are circular molecules of DNA. In the mouse fibroblast cell line, 3T3DM, the double minute chromosomes include the Mdm2 gene on a 4-Mb circle and two identical inverted repeat molecules that are linked by spacer molecules of heterogeneous size.[105]

Chemical mutagenesis. The rate of mutation for individual genes in human somatic cells has been measured to be about 10^{-7} to about 10^{-8} for HLA and glycophorin A.[106,107] These rates of mutation are determined by exposure to free radicals of oxygen, the inherent rates of deamination and depurivation of DNA, and by replication errors. It has been calculated that the rates of free-radical disruption of DNA and depurinations are both on the order of 10^4 per cell per day.[108] The observed mutational frequency represents that proportion of mutagenic events that are not repaired by endogenous mechanisms.

Chemical agents can enhance the rate of mutation in human cells. These agents can cause depurination, deamination of 5-methylcytosine, and oxidative damage from free radicals.[109] A common mechanism of these agents is electrophilic attack of DNA bases. During DNA replication, the chemically adducted site is repaired, but not back to the original base. The altered base is then transmitted to progeny cells.

Each mutagenic agent produces characteristic alterations at specific locations in DNA, so-called "fingerprints." Aflatoxin B_1 is a potent liver carcinogen that is found in fungal-contaminated grains in Qiday in regions of China and southern Africa. This agent forms N^7-deoxyguanosine adducts that lead to base substitutions, principally G-to-T transversions. A high proportion of hepatocellular carcinomas from China and southern Africa were found to have G-to-T mutations at codon 249 of the p53 gene.[110,111] This molecular fingerprint was not observed in the p53 genes of hepatocellular carcinomas from Chinese in Singapore, a place that is not endemic for aflatoxin B_1.[112]

Many chemical agents require metabolic activation to exert carcinogenic effects. Quantitative differences in carcinogen metabolism and in the formation of carcinogen–DNA adducts occur between individuals as well as among different cell and tissue types of a given individual.[113] These quantitative differences may influence an individual's risk for developing cancer as well as the tissue site at which cancer may occur.

Many of the enzymes that catalyze metabolic activation are members of the cytochrome P-450 family.[114] The activity of these enzymes can vary several-thousand-fold, and the more active enzyme forms are associated with increased cancer risk. The active hydroxylator phenotype of the cytochrome P-450, CYP2D6, has been associated with an eightfold increase in risk for lung cancers (other than adenocarcinomas) compared to the poor hydroxylator phenotype.[114] This enzyme hydroxylates N-nitrosamine in tobacco, a potential carcinogen.

Hypermutation in immunoglobulin genes. The initial antibody response is mounted by light- and heavy-chain subunits that are assembled in the rough endoplasmic reticulum of B lymphocytes.[115] These subunits are synthesized from immunoglobulin light-chain and heavy-chain genes that have undergone recombination. Recombination occurs between the variable (V), joining (J), and constant (C) regions of the immunoglobulin κ light-chain genes on chromosome 2 and immunoglobulin λ light-chain genes on chromosome 22.[116–119] Specific recombination signal sequences include a dyad-symmetric hepatamer sequence directly adjacent to the coding region and an AT-rich nonamer sequence that is separated from the hepatamer by a spacer region of nonconserved nucleotides.[120–121] These sites are recognized by a genetically encoded recombinase that mediates the recombinational process.[123,124]

Similar regions exist for the immunoglobulin heavy-chain genes on chromosome 14.[125] An additional region, termed D for "diversity," is located between the J and C regions.[126] Different constant regions are genetically encoded and determine the specificity of the immunoglobulin molecules, whether the immunoglobulin is maintained on the cell surface or secreted, and whether the antibody is part of a primary, secondary, or allergic immune response.[127]

A second form of mutation in immunoglobulin genes is termed *junctional diversity*. During the process of recombination, the joining of ends is imprecise.[128,129] Both loss and gain of bases occur. Random addition of nucleotides at the coding junctions of immunoglobulin may be mediated by the enzyme terminal deoxynucleotidyl transferase (TdT).[130] This enzyme has a preference for G nucleotides but will insert any at the 3' ends of DNA molecules without a template present. The resulting single-stranded 3' additions may be joined by the recombinase and then be repaired by other DNA polymerases.

An additional level of specificity in the immune response occurs as the result of somatic hypermutation in the recombined immunoglobulin genes. High rates of mutation occur in immunoglobulin genes even in the absence of malignancy or a generalized mutator phenotype.[131] As the B cells proliferate in the germinal centers, replication errors are made in the rearranged V genes. The rate of mutation is 10^{-4}–10^{-3} per base per replication event, suggesting that replication repair is less faithful in mature B cells for errors in this region of the gene.[132,133] Alternatively, it has been proposed that the hypermutation is directly related to transcription of the immunoglobulin gene.[134] Errors are introduced into the sequence during transcription and during the formation of a reverse transcriptase DNA copy. The mutated cDNA intermediate is either integrated into the normal chromosome site by gene conversion or subject to additional cycles of error-prone transcription/reverse transcription on an episome prior to reintegration. B cells with somatic mutation events that result in the production of higher-affinity antibodies are selected for and proliferate.[135]

Somatic hypermutation is likely to play a role in autoimmune diseases, such as rheumatoid arthritis and systemic lupus erythematosus. Efforts to identify a specific group of V genes that are associated with autoimmune disorders have been by and large unsuccessful. The rheumatoid factors that make up the antibodies in rheumatoid arthritis are derived from a diverse array of V gene segments even for a single individual.[136] Four cell lines that made high-affinity rheumatoid factors from a patient with rheumatoid arthritis used different V and J gene segments but demonstrated somatic hypermutation.[137] Thus, it appears that production of autoantibodies in autoimmune diseases represents a combination of somatic hypermutation coupled to a loss of normal regulation, leading to overproduction of these antibodies.

In germ cells, rates of mutation and recombination alter the phenotype of the progeny compared to their parents. These events may be recognized as anticipation of that disorder in a family. In somatic cells, high rates of mutation alter the phenotype of the individuals over time. Some events, such as malignancy or occurrence of multiple malformations, may be the effect of a mutator phenotype. Other events, such as production of immunoglobulins, are physiologic. Because some somatic changes alter the ability of the individual to respond to external stimuli over time, they undoubtedly play a role in disease and in the aging process.

These processes reflect the genetic properties of each individual; however, new genetic information may be incorporated into somatic cells and germ cells by endogenous genetic elements. These elements are contained by viruses, naked strands of DNA, and proteinaceous particles that spend part of their life cycle in one person, are shed, and then are taken up by another person.

REFERENCES

1. Pembrey ME, Winter RM, Davies KE. A premutation that generates a defect at crossing over explains the inheritance of fragile X mental retardation. Am J Med Genet 21:709–717, 1985.
2. Nussbaum RL, Ledbetter DH. Fragile X syndrome: a unique mutation in man. Annu Rev Genet 20:109–145, 1986.
3. Mott FW. A lecture on heredity and insanity. Lancet 1:1251–1259, 1911.
4. Penrose LS. The problem of anticipation in pedigrees of dystrophic myotonica. Ann Eugen 14:125–132, 1948.
5. Howeler CJ, Bush HFM, Geraedts JPM, Niermeijer MF, Stall A. Anticipation in myotonic dystrophy: fact or fiction. Brain 12:779–797, 1989.
6. Bell J. On the age of onset and age at death in hereditary muscular dystrophy with some observations bearing on the question of antedating. Ann Eugen 11:272–289, 1942.
7. Harper PS, Harley HG, Reardon W, Shaw DJ. Anticipation in myotonic dystrophy: new light on an old problem. Am J Hum Genet 51:10–16, 1992.
8. Harper PS. Myotonic Dystrophy. Philadelphia: WB Saunders, 1989.
9. Fleischer B. Uber myuotonische Dystrophie mit Katarakt. Albrecht von Graefes Arch Klin Exp Ophthalmol 96:91–133, 1918.
10. Harper PS, Dyken PR. Early-onset dystrophia myotonica: evidence supporting a maternal environmental factor. Lancet 2:53–55, 1972.
11. Koch MC, Grimm T, Harley HG, Harper PS. Genetic risks for children of women with myotonic dystrophy. Am J Hum Genet 48:1084–1091, 1991.
12. Martin JP, Bell J. A pedigree of mental defect showing sex-linkage. J Neurol Psychiatr 6:154–157, 1943.
13. Lubs HA, Jr. A marker X chromosome. Am J Hum Genet 21:231–244, 1969.
14. Sherman SL, Jacobs PA, Morton NE, Froster-Iskenius U, Howard-Peebles PN, Nielsen KB, et al. Further segregation analysis of the fragile X syndrome with special reference to transmitting males. Hum Genet 69:289–299, 1985.

15. Sherman SL, Morton NE, Jacobs PA, Turner G. The marker (X) syndrome: a cyto-genetic and genetic analysis. Ann Hum Genet 48:21–37, 1984.

16. Nussbaum RL, Airhart SD, Ledbetter DH. Recombination and amplification of pyrimidine-rich sequences may be responsible for initiation and progression of the Xq27 fragile site: a hypothesis. Am J Med Genet 23:715–722, 1986.

17. Fu YH, Kuhl DP, Pizzuti A, Pieretti M, Sutcliffe JS, Richards S, et al. Variation of the CGG repeat at the fragile X site results in genetic instability: resolution of the Sherman paradox. Cell 67:1047–1058, 1991.

18. Yu S, Pritchard M, Kremer E, Lynch M, Nancarrow J, Baker K, et al. Fragile X genotype characterized by an unstable region of DNA. Science 252:1179–11819, 1991.

19. Verkerk AJMH, Pieretti M, Sutcliffe JS, Fu YH, Kuhl DPA, Pizzuti A, et al. Identi-fication of a gene (FMR-1) containing a CGG repeat coincident with a breakpoint cluster region exhibiting length variation in fragile X syndrome. Cell 65:905–914, 1991.

20. Heitz D, Devys D, Imbert G, Kretz C, Mandel JL. Inheritance of the fragile X syndrome: size of the fragile X premutation is a major determinant of the transition to full mutation. J Med Genet 29:794–801, 1992.

21. Eichler EE, Holden JJ, Popovich BW, Reiss AL, Snow K, Thibodeau SN, et al. Length of uninterrupted CGG repeats determines instability in the FMR1. Nat Genet 8:88–94, 1994.

22. Chakravarti A. Fragile X founder effect? Nat Genet 1:237–238, 1992.

23. Richards RI, Holman K, Friend K, Kremer E, Hillen D, Staples A, et al. Evidence of founder chromosomes in fragile X. Nat Genet 1:257–260, 1992.

24. Reyniers E, Vits L, De Boulle K, Van Roy B, Van Velzen D, de Graaff E, et al. The full mutation in the FMR-1 gene of male fragile X patients is absent in their sperm. Nat Genet 4:143–148, 1993.

25. Brook JD, McCurrach ME, Harley HG, Buckler AJ, Church D, Aburatani H, et al. Molecular basis of myotonic dystrophy: expansion of a trinucleotide (CTG) repeat at the 3' end of a transcript encoding a protein kinase family member. Cell 68:799–808, 1992.

26. Mahadevan M, Tsilfidis C, Sabourin L, Shutler G, Amemiya C, Jansen G, et al. Myotonic dystrophy mutation: an unstable CTG repeat in the 3' untranslated region of the gene. Science 255:1253–1255, 1992.

27. Aslanidis C, Jansen G, Amemiya C, Shutler G, Mahadevan M, Tsilfidis C, et al. Cloning of the essential myotonic dystrophy region and mapping of the putative defect. Nature 355:548–551, 1992.

28. Harley HG, Brook JD, Rundle SA, Crow S, Reardon W, Buckler AJ, et al. Expan-sion of an unstable DNA region and phenotypic variation in myotonic dystrophy. Nature 355:545–546, 1992.

29. Tsilfidis C, MacKenzie AE, Mettler G, Barcelo J, Korneluk RG. Correlation of CTG trinucleotide repeat length and frequency of severe congenital myotonic dystrophy. Nat Genet 1:192–195, 1992.

30. Brunner H, Smeets H, Coerwinkel-Driessen M, van Oost BA, Spaans F, Wieringa B, et al. Influence of sex of the transmitting parent as well as of parental allele size on the CTG expansion in myotonic dystrophy (DM). Am J Hum Genet 53:1016–1023, 1993.

31. Harley HG, Brook JD, Floyd J, Rundle SA, Crow S, Walsh KV, et al. Detection of linkage disequilibrium between the myotonic dystrophy locus and a new polymor-phic DNA marker. Am J Hum Genet 49:68–75, 1991.

32. MacKenzie AE, MacLeod HL, Hunter AGW, Korneluk RG. Linkage analysis of the Apolipoprotein C2 gene and myotonic dystrophy on human chromosome 19 reveals linkage disequilibrium in a French-Canadian population. Am J Hum Genet 44:140–147, 1989.

33. The Huntington's Disease Collaborative Research Group. A novel gene containing a trinucleotide repeat that is expanded and unstable on Huntington's disease chromosomes. Cell 72:971–983, 1993.

34. Orr HT, Chung M, Banfi S, Kwiatkowski, Jr., Servadio A, Beaudet AL, et al. Expansion of an unstable trinucleotide CAG repeat in spinocerebellar ataxia type 1. Nat Genet 4:221–226, 1993.

35. Banfi S, Servadio A, Chung M, Kwiatkowski, Jr., McCall AE, Duvick LA, et al. Identification and characterization of the gene causing type 1 spinocerebellar ataxia. Nat Genet 7:513–519, 1994.

36. Kawaguchi Y, Okamoto T, Taniwaki M, Aizawa M, Inoue M, Katayama S, et al. CAG expansions in a novel gene for Marchado-Joseph disease at chromosome 14q32.1. Nat Genet 8:221–228, 1994.

37. Nagafuchi S, Yanagisawa H, Sato K, Shirayama T, Osaki E, Bundo M, et al. Dentatorubral and pallidolusian atrophy expansion of an unstable CAG trinucleotide on chromosome 12p. Nat Genet 6:14–18, 1994.

38. Koide R, Ikeuchi T, Onodera O, Tanaka H, Igarashi S, Endo K, et al. Unstable expansion of CAG repeat in hereditary dentatorubral-pallidolusian atrophy (DRPLA). Nat Genet 6:9–13, 1994.

39. Pulst S-M, Nechiporuk A, Nechiporuk T, Gispert S, Chen X-N, Lopes-Cendes I, et al. Moderate expansion of a normal biallelic trinucleotide repeat in spinocerebellar ataxia type 2. Nat Genet 14:269–276, 1996.

40. Hayden MR. Huntington's Chorea. Berlin: Springer-Verlag, 1981.

41. Myers RH, Madden JJ, Teague JL, Falek A. Factors related to onset age of Huntington disease. Am J Hum Genet 34:481–488, 1982.

42. Brackenridge CJ. The relation of type of initial symptoms and line of transmission to ages at onset and death in Huntington's disease. Clin Genet 2:287–297, 1971.

43. Ambrose CM, Duyao MP, Barnes G, Bate GP, Lin CS, Srinidhi J, et al. Structure and expression of the Huntington's disease gene: evidence against simple inactivation due to an expanded CAG repeat. Somat Cell Mol Genet 20:27–38, 1994.

44. Rubinsztein DC, Barton DE, Davidson BCC, Ferguson-Smith MA. Analysis of the huntington gene reveals a trinucleotide-length polymorphism in the region of the gene that contains two CCG-rich stretches and a correlation between decreased age of onset of Huntington's disease and CAG repeat number. Hum Mol Genet 2:1713–1715, 1993.

45. Zoghbi HY, Pollack MS, Lyons LA, Ferrell RE, Daigner SP, Beaudet AL. Spinocerebellar ataxia; variable age of onset and linkage to HLA in a large kindred. Ann Neurol 23:580–584, 1988.

46. Naito H, Oyanagi S. Familial myoclonus epilepsy and choreoathetosis: hereditary dentatorubral-pallidolusian atrophy. Neurology 32:798–807, 1982.

47. La Spada AR, Wilson WM, Lubahn DB, Harding AE, Fischbeck KH. Androgen receptor gene mutations in X-linked spinal and bulbar muscle atrophy. Nature 352:77–79, 1991.

48. Knight SJL, Flannery AV, Hirst MC, Campbell L, Christodoulou Z, Phelps SR, et al. Trinucleotide repeat amplification and hypermethylation of a CpG island in FRAXE mental retardation. Cell 74:127–134, 1993.

49. Kennedy WR, Alter M, Sung JH. Progressive proximal spinal and bulbar muscular atrophy of late onset: a sex-linked recessive trait. Neurology 18:671–680, 1968.

50. Sutherland GR, Baker E. Characterization of a new rare fragile site easily confused with the fragile X. Hum Mol Genet 1:111–113, 1992.

51. Margolis RL, Breschel TS, Li SH, Kidwai AS, Antonarakis SE, McInnes MG, et al. Characterization of cDNA clones containing CCA trinucleotide repeats derived from human brain. Somat Cell Mol Genet 21:279–284, 1995.

52. Margolis RL, Breschel TS, Li SH, Kidwai AS, McInnis MG, Ross CA. Polymorphic (AAT) in trinucleotide repeats derived from a human brain cDNA library. Hum Genet 96:495–496, 1995.

53. Gubbay J, Collignon J, Koopman P, Capel B, Economou A, Munsterberg A, et al. A gene mapping to the sex-determining region of the mouse Y chromosome is a member of a novel family of embryonically expressed genes. Nature 346:245–250, 1990.

54. Dubin RA, Ostrer H. Sry is a transcriptional activator. Mol Endocrinol 8:1182–1192, 1994.

55. Stark GR, Wahl GM. Gene amplification. Annu Rev Biochem 53:447–491, 1984.

56. Martorell L, Martinez JM, Carey N, Johnson K, Baiget M. Comparison of CTG repeat length expansion and clinical progression of myotonic dystrophy over a five year period. J Med Genet 32:593–596, 1995.

57. Cross SH, Allshire RC, McKay SJ, McGill NI, Cooke HJ. Cloning of human telomeres by complementation in yeast. Nature 338:771–774, 1989.

58. Harley CB, Futcher AB, Greider CW. Telomeres shorten during ageing of human fibroblasts. Nature 345:458–460, 1990.

59. Morin GB. The human telomere terminal transferase enzyme is a ribonucleoprotein that synthesizes TTAGGG repeats. Cell 59:521–529, 1989.

60. Hastie ND, Dempster M, Dunlop MG, Thompson AM, Green DK, Allshire RC. Telomere reduction in human colorectal carcinoma and with ageing. Nature 346:866–868, 1990.

61. Morin GB. Recognition of a chromosome truncation site associated with alpha-thalassaemia by human telomerase. Nature 353:454–456, 1991.

62. Vaziri H, Schachter F, Uchida I, Wei L, Zhu X, Effros R, et al. Loss of telomeric DNA during aging of normal and trisomy 21 human lymphocytes. Am J Hum Genet 52:661–667, 1993.

63. Hayflick L. The limited in vitro lifetime of human diploid cell strains. Exp Cell Res 37:614–636, 1965.

64. Lynch HT, Mulcahy GM, Harris RE, Guirgis HA, Lynch JF. Genetic and pathologic findings in a kindred with hereditary sarcoma breast cancer, brain tumors, leukemia, lung, laryngeal, and adrenal cortical carcinoma. Cancer 41:2055–2064, 1978.

65. Aaltonen LA, Peltomaki P, Leach FS, Sistonen P, Pylkkanen L, Mecklin J-P, et al. Clues to the pathogenesis of familial colorectal cancer. Science 260:812–816, 1993.

66. Fishel R, Lescoe MK, Rao MRS, Copeland NG, Jenkins NA, Garber J, et al. The human mutator gene homolog MSH2 and its association with hereditary nonpolyposis colon cancer. Cell 75:1027–1038, 1993.

67. Leach FS, Nicolaides NC, Papadopoulos N, Liu B, Jen J, Parsons R, et al. Mutations of a MutS homolog in hereditary non-polyposis colorectal cancer. Cell 75:1215–1225, 1993.

68. Papadopoulos N, Nicolaides NC, Wei Y-F, Ruben SM, Carter KC, Rosen CA, et al. Mutation of a mutL homolog in hereditary colon cancer. Science 263:1625–1629, 1994.

69. Bronner CE, Baker SM, Morrison PT, Warren G, Smith LG, Loscoe MK, et al. Mutation in the DNA mismatch repair gene homologue hMLH1 is associated with hereditary non-polyposis colon cancer. Nature 368:258–261, 1994.

70. Nicolaides NC, Papadopoulos N, Liu B, Wei Y-F, Carter KC, Ruben SM, et al. Mutations of two PMS homologues in hereditary nonpolyposis colon cancer. Nature 371:75–80, 1994.

71. Modrich P, Mismatch repair, genetic stability and cancer. Science 266:1959–60, 1994.

72. Parsons R, Li G-M, Longley MJ, Fang WH, Papadopoulos N, Jen J, et al. Hypermutability and mismatch repair deficiency in RER(+) tumor cells. Cell 75:1227–1236, 1993.

73. Cleaver JE. Xeroderma pigmentosum: biochemical and genetic characteristics. Annu Rev Genet 9:19–38, 1975.

74. Cleaver JE. Defective repair replication of DNA in xeroderma pigmentosum. Nature 218:652–656, 1968.

75. Goldstein S, Lin CC. Survival and DNA repair of somatic cell hybrids after ultraviolet irradiation. Nature 239:142–145, 1972.

76. Bootsma D, Hoeijmakers JHJ. The genetic basis of xeroderma pigmentosum. Ann Genet 34:143–150, 1991.

77. Tanaka K, Miura N, Satokata I, Miyamoto I, Yoshida MC, Satoh Y, et al. Analysis of a human DNA excision repair gene involved in group A xeroderma pigmentosum and containing a zinc-finger domain. Nature 348:73–76, 1990.

78. Weeda G, van Ham RCA, Vermeulen W, Bootsma D, van der Eb AJ, Hoeijmakers JHJ. A presumed DNA helicase encoded by ERCC-3 is involved in the human repair disorders xeroderma pigmentosum and Cockayne's syndrome. Cell 62:777–791, 1990.

79. Flejter WL, McDaniel LD, Johns D, Friedberg EC, Schultz RA. Correction of xeroderma pigmentosum complementation group D mutant cell phenotypes by chromosome and gene transfer: involvement of the human ERCC2 DNA repair gene. Proc Natl Acad Sci 89:261–265, 1992.

80. Sijbers AM, de Laat WL, Ariza RR, Biggerstaff M, Wei Y-F, Moggs JG, et al. Xeroderma pigmentosum group F caused by a defect in a structure-specific DNA repair endonuclease. Dell 86:811–822, 1996.

81. O'Donovan A, Scherly D, Clarkson SG, Wood RD. Isolation of active recombinant XPG protein, a human DNA repair endonuclease. J Biol Chem 269:15965–15968, 1994.

82. Schroeder TM, German JB. Bloom's syndrome and Fanconi's anemia: demonstration of two distinctive patterns of chromosome disruption and rearrangement. Humangenetik 25:299–306, 1974.

83. Garriga S, Crosby WH. The incidence of leukemia in families of patients with hypoplasia of the marrow. Blood 14:1008–1014, 1959.

84. Giampietro PF, Adler-Brecher B, Verlander PC, Pavlakis SG, Davis JG, Auerbach AD. The need for more accurate and timely diagnosis in Fanconi anemia: a report from the International Fanconi Anemia Registry. Pediatrics 91:1116–1120, 1993.

85. Dutrillaux B, Autias A, Dutrillaux A-M, Buriot D, Prieur M. The cell cycle of lymphocytes in Fanconi anemia. Hum Genet 62:327–332, 1982.

86. Auerbach AD, Rogatko A, Schroeder-Kurth TM. International Fanconi Anemia Registry: relation of clinical symptoms to diepoxybutane sensitivity. Blood 73:391–396, 1989.

87. Fanconi Anaemia/Breast Cancer Consortium. Positional cloning of the Fanconi anaemia group A gene. Nat Genet 14:324–328, 1996.

88. Strathdee CA, Gavish H, Shannon WR, Buchwald M. Cloning of cDNAs for Fanconi's anaemia by functional complementation. Nature 356:763–767, 1992.

89. Bloom D. The syndrome of congenital telangiectatic erythema and stunted growth. J Pediatr 68:103–113, 1966.

90. Ellis NA, Lennon DJ, Proytcheva M, Alhadeff B, Henderson EE, German J. Somatic intragenic recombination within the mutated locus BLM can correct the high SCE phenotype of Bloom syndrome cells. Am J Hum Genet 57:1019–1027, 1995.

91. Ellis NA, Groden J, Ye T-Z, Straughen J, Lennon DJ, Ciocci S, et al. The Bloom's syndrome gene product is homologous to RecQ helicases. Cell 83:655–666, 1995.

92. Gatti RA, Swift M. Ataxia-telangiectasia: Genetics, Neuropathology, and Immunology of a Degenerative Disease of Childhood. New York: Alan R Liss, 1985.

93. Oxford JM, Harnden DG, Parrington JM, Delhanty JDA. Specific chromosome aberrations in ataxia-telangiectasia. J Med Genet 12:251–262, 1975.

94. Painter RB, Young BR. Radiosensitivity in ataxia-telangiectasia: a new explanation. Proc Natl Acad Sci USA 77:7315–7317, 1980.

95. Swift M, Reitnauer PJ, Morrell D, Chase CL. Breast and other cancers in families with ataxia-telangiectasia. N Engl J Med 316:1289–1294, 1987.

96. Slamon DJ, Godolphin W, Jones LA, Holt JA, Wong SG, Keith DE, et al. Studies of the HER-2/neu proto-oncogene in human breast and ovarian cancer. Science 244:707–712, 1989.

97. Schwab M, Ellison J, Busch M, Rosenau W, Varmus HE, Bishop JM. Enhanced expression of the human gene N-myc consequent to amplification of DNA may contribute to malignant progression of neuroblastoma. Proc Natl Acad Sci USA 81:4940–4944, 1984.

98. Riordan JR, Deuchars K, Kartner N, Alon N, Trent J, Ling V. Amplification of P-glycoprotein genes in multidrug-resistant mammalian cell lines. Nature 316:817–819, 1985.

99. Momand J, Zambetti GP, Olson DC, George D, Levine AJ. The mdm-2 oncogene product forms a complex with the p53 protein and inhibits p53-mediated transactivation. Cell 69:1237–1245, 1992.

100. Khatib ZA, Matsushime H, Valentine M, Shapiro DN, Sherr CJ, Look AT. Coamplification of the CDK4 gene with MDM2 and GLI in human sarcomas. Cancer Res 53:5535–5541, 1993.

101. Tam SW, Theodoras AM, Shay JW, Draetta GF, Pagano M. Differential expression and regulation of cyclin D1 protein in normal and tumor human cells: association with Cdk4 is required for cyclin D1 function in G1 progression. Oncogene 9:2663–2674, 1994.

102. Kinzler KW, Vogelstein B. The GLI gene encodes a nuclear protein which binds specific sequences in the human genome. Mol Cell Biol 10:634–642, 1990.

103. Von Hoff DD, Needham-VanDevanter DR, Yucel J, Windle BE, Wahl GM. Amplified human MYC oncogenes localized to replicating submicroscopic circular DNA molecules. Proc Natl Acad Sci USA 85:4804–4808, 1988.

104. Balaban-Malenbaum G, Gilbert F. Double minute chromosomes and the homogeneously staining regions in chromosomes of a human neuroblastoma cell line. Science 198:739–741, 1977.

105. Fakjarzadeh SS, Rosenblum-Vos L, Murphy M, Hoffman EK, George DL. Structure and organization of amplified DNA on double minutes containing the mdm2 oncogene. Genomics 15:283–290, 1993.

106. Langlois RG, Bigbee WL, Jensen RH. Measurements of the frequency of human erythrocytes with gene expression loss phenotypes at the glycophorin A locus. Hum Genet 74:353–362, 1986.

107. Pious D, Soderland C. HLA variants of cultured human lymphoid cells: evidence for mutational origin and estimation of mutation rate. Science 197:769–771, 1977.

108. Loeb LA, Cheng KC. Errors in DNA synthesis: a source of spontaneous mutations. Mutat Res 238:297–304, 1990.

109. Lehmann AR, Hoeijmakers JH, van Zeeland AA, Backendorf CM, Bridges BA, Collins A, et al. Workshop on DNA repair. Mutat Res 273:1–28, 1992.

110. Hsu IC, Metcalf RA, Sun T, Welsh JA, Wang NJ, Harris CC. Mutational hotspot in the p53 gene in human hepatocellular carcinomas. Nature 350:427–428, 1991.

111. Aguilar F, Harris CC, Sun T, Hollstein M, Cerutti P. Geographic variation of p53 mutational profile in nonmalignant human liver. Science 264:1317–1319, 1994.

112. Shi CY, Phang TW, Lin Y, Wee A, Li B, Lee HP, et al. Codon 249 mutation of the p53 gene is a rare event in hepatocellular carcinomas from ethnic Chinese in Singapore. Br J Cancer 72:146–149, 1995.

113. Guengerich FP, Distlerath LM, Reilly PEB, Wolff T, Shimada T, Umbenhauer DR, et al. Human liver cytochromes P-450 involved in polymorphisms of drug oxidation. Xenobiotica 16:367–378, 1986.

114. Sugimura H, Caporaso NE, Shaw GL, Modali RV, Gonzalez FJ, Hoover RN, et al. Human debrisoquine hydroxylase gene polymorphisms in cancer patients and controls. Carcinogenesis 11:1527–1530, 1990.

115. Askonas BA. Immunoglobulin formation in B lymphoid cells. J Clin Pathol 6:8–12, 1975.

116. Hieter PA, Maizel JV, Jr., Leder P. Evolution of human immunoglobulin kappa J region genes. J Biol Chem 257:1516–1522, 1982.

117. Hieter PA, Max EE, Seidman JG, Maizel JV, Jr., Leder P. Cloned human and mouse kappa immunoglubulin constant and J region genes conserve homology in functional segments. Cell 22:197–207, 1980.

118. Malcolm S, Barton P, Murphy C, Ferguson-Smith MA, Bentley DL. Localization of human immunoglubulin kappa light chain variable region genes to the short arm of chromosome 2 by in situ hybridization. Proc Natl Acad Sci USA 79:4957–4961, 1982.

119. Erikson J, Martinis J, Croce CM. Assignment of the genes for human lambda immunoglobulin chains to chromosome 22. Nature 294:173–175, 1981.

120. Max EE, Seidman JG, Leder P. Sequences of five potential recombination sites encoded close to an immunoglobulin kappa constant region gene. Proc Natl Acad Sci USA 76:3450–3454, 1979.

121. Sakano H, Huppi K, Heinrich G, Tonegawa S. Sequences at the somatic recombination sites of immunoglobulin light-chain genes. Nature 280:288–294, 1979.

122. Bernard O, Hozumi N, Tonegawa S. Sequences of mouse immunoglobulin light chain genes before and after somatic changes. Cell 15:1133–1144, 1978.

123. Schatz DG, Oettinger MA, Baltimore D. The V(D)J recombination activating gene, RAG-1. Cell 59:1035–1048, 1989.

124. Oettinger MA, Schatz DG, Gorka C, Baltimore D. RAG-1 and RAG-2, adjacent genes that synergistically activate V(D)J recombination. Science 248:1517–1523, 1990.

125. McBride OW, Battey J, Hollis GF, Swan DC, Siebenlist U, Leder P. Localization of human variable and constant region immunoglobulin heavy chain genes on subtelomeric band q32 of chromosome 14. Nucleic Acids Res 10:8155–8170, 1982.

126. Ravetch JV, Siebenlist U, Korsmeyer S, Waldmann T, Leder P. Structure of the human immunoglobulin mu locus: characterization of embryonic and rearranged J and D genes. Cell 27:583–591, 1981.

127. Ravetch JV, Kirsch IR, Leder P. Evolutionary approach to the question of immunoglobulin heavy chain switching: evidence from cloned human and mouse genes. Proc Natl Acad Sci USA 77:6734–6738, 1980.

128. Pollok BA, Kearney JF, Vakil M, Perry RP. A biological consequence of variation in the site of D-JH gene rearrangement. Nature 311:376–379, 1984.

129. Jeske DJ, Jarvis J, Milstein C, Capra JD. Junctional diversity is essential to antibody activity. J Immunol 133:1090–1092, 1984.

130. Desiderio SV, Yancopoulos GD, Paskind M, Thomas E, Boss MA, Landau N, et al. Insertion of N regions into heavy-chain genes is correlated with expression of terminal deoxytransferase in B cells. Nature 311:752–755, 1984.

131. Allen D, Cumano A, Dildrop R, Kocks C, Rajewsky K, Rajewsky N, et al. Timing, genetic requirements and functional consequences of somatic hypermutation during B-cell development. Immunol Rev 96:5–22, 1987.

132. Rogerson B, Hackett J, Peters A, Haasch D, Storb U. Mutation pattern of immunoglobulin transgenes is compatible with a model of somatic hypermutation in which targeting of the mutator is linked to the direction of DNA replication. EMBO J 10:4331–4341, 1991.

133. Jolly CJ, Wagner SD, Rada C, Klix N, Milstein C, Neuberger MS. The targeting of somatic hypermutation. Semin Immunol 8:159–168, 1996.

134. Storb U, Peters A, Klotz E, Rogerson B, Hackett J, Jr. The mechanism of somatic hypermutation studied with transgenic and transfected target genes. Semin Immunol 8:131–140, 1996.

135. Fairhurst RM, Valles-Ayoub Y, Neshat M, Braun J. A DNA repair abnormality specific for rearranged immunoglobulin variable genes in germinal center B cells. Mol Immunol 33:231–244, 1996.

136. Fang Q, Kannapell CC, Gaskin F, Solomon A, Koopman WJ, Fu SM. Human rheumatoid factors with restrictive specificity for rabbit immunoglobulin G: auto- and multireactivity, diverse VH gene segment usage and preferential usage of V lambda IIIb. J Exp Med 179:1445–1456, 1994.

137. Mantovani L, Wilder RL, Casali P. Human rheumatoid B-1a (CD5 + B) cells make somatically hypermutated high affinity IgM rheumatoid factors. J Immunol 151:473–488, 1993.

9
Viral Infection

Infection by viruses can cause human somatic cells to undergo transient or stable genetic changes. Once inside the cell, the viral nucleic acid may integrate into the host genome or may remain in the unincorporated state. The virus may use host proteins to replicate and package their own genomes and the products of the host's metabolism as sources of energy. Through their interactions with infected cells, viruses may alter the phenotype of the cell, producing a direct cytotoxic effect, an inflammatory response, or a selective growth advantage. Some viruses may act as true endosymbionts, producing no pathologic effects at all.

Some viruses that use humans as their reservoir may demonstrate a pattern of transmission that may simulate genetic inheritance. This pattern of inheritance may be from parent to child (vertical), among siblings (horizontal), among sons or daughters only (sex-linked), and may skip generations. Infected members of a family may manifest symptoms at the same time or at different times or may have recurring symptoms. The symptoms may be similar or highly divergent among infected individuals *(pleiotropy)*. Different agents may produce similar symptoms or may even mimic Mendelian genetic conditions *(phenocopies)*.

Ironically, despite the fact that viral infection is the prototype of an environmental agent for causing disease, viruses may use many of the same disease-causing mechanisms as mutated cellular genes. The similarities between viral genes and host genes are striking. Both rely on the relatively stable transmission of genetic information. Both make use of cellular mechanisms of replication.

169

THE LIFE CYCLE OF HUMAN VIRUSES

Extracellular phase. Human viruses have an extracellular phase to their life cycle, making them exogenous agents (Fig. 9.1).[1–8] The viral genome is comprised of either DNA or RNA. During the extracellular phase, the viral genome is surrounded by a protein shell, or *capsid.* The capsid is comprised of one or more protein subunits that are encoded by the viral genome. The associated nucleic acid and capsid together are termed *nucleocapsid.* Many viruses have an additional lipid membrane envelope that is acquired as the viral nucleocapsid buds through the cell membrane. The capsid and envelope are instrumental for conferring stability and for determining the infectivity of the agent. Capsid proteins and proteins inserted in the lipid membrane form specific associations with receptors of the host cells. For example, the CD4 T-cell antigen is the receptor for the human immunodeficiency viruses, and the type 2 complement receptor on B cells, CD21, is the receptor for the Epstein-Barr virus.[9,10]

Some agents, such as poxviruses, are resistant to drying and retain their stability for many years when free from the intracellular environment of the host.[1] Their resistance to drying and heat is determined by the structure of their genomes and their surrounding capsids and envelopes. Some agents, such as the human immunodeficiency viruses (HIV1 and HIV2), do not resist drying and are transmitted only by direct transmission of bodily fluids.[11]

Infectious agents vary in their sensitivity to ultraviolet light. Generally this reflects the formation of thymine dimers that may introduce lethal mutations.[12] *Prions* or slow viruses (so-called because they take years to manifest their phenotypic effects) are thought to be devoid of nucleic acids or to have small nucleic acid genomes because they are relatively resistant to the effects of ultraviolet light.[13,14]

Infection. The viral particle is absorbed onto a receptor and then moves into a specialized region of the cell membrane known as a *coated pit* (Fig. 9.1).[15] The plasma membrane engulfs the particle, then buds off and transports the

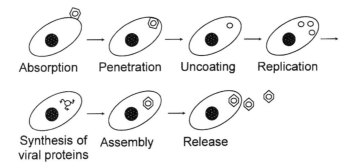

Absorption   Penetration   Uncoating   Replication

Synthesis of   Assembly   Release
viral proteins

Figure 9.1. Idealized life cycle of viruses in infected cells. The steps include absorption, penetration, uncoating, replication, synthesis of viral proteins, assembly, and release.

particle into the cell.[16] The transport vesicle fuses with an endosome in the interior of the cell. The viral envelope, if present, fuses with that of the endosome. The viral particle is partially or completely uncoated. Once uncoated, the viral genome may be transported to the cell nucleus. Alternatively, it may remain in the cytoplasm, where it replicates (Fig. 9.2).

The genetic information of RNA-containing viruses is expressed soon after uncoating. For DNA-containing viruses, the life cycle can be divided into early and late periods.[1,3–8] Steps during the early phase include (1) inhibition of host DNA, RNA, and protein synthesis, causing viral rather than host genetic information to be processed, (2) the synthesis of proteins that form the matrix for viral nucleic acid replication and viral morphogenesis, and (3) the synthesis of viral DNA and RNA polymerases.

During the late phase of viral replication, genes are expressed for viral structural proteins, enzymes, and other components that function in viral particle assembly. The assembly process is spontaneous, and the information for assembly resides in the amino acid sequences of the capsid proteins.[2,17,18] Nucleic acids do not play an essential role in assembly but are packaged into the assembled particles.

The last step in the viral replication cycle is the release of progeny particles. Unenveloped viruses are released when the host cells disintegrate. This may simply reflect that infected cells may disintegrate more rapidly than uninfected cells. For enveloped viruses, release is the final stage of morphogenesis. Viral proteins are incorporated into certain areas of the host cell membrane. The

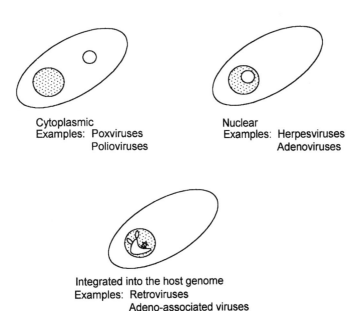

Cytoplasmic
Examples: Poxviruses
        Polioviruses

Nuclear
Examples: Herpesviruses
        Adenoviruses

Integrated into the host genome
Examples: Retroviruses
        Adeno-associated viruses

Figure 9.2. Localization of viral genomes in infected cells. Viral proteins may be cytoplasmic or nuclear in their location and may integrate into the host genome.

nucleocapsids are built onto these proteins. The nucleocapsids then bud through the membrane patches, creating a free, but enveloped, membrane particle.[19]

Latency. A virus may remain latent, a state in which it replicates its genome but does not produce infectious particles.[20–23] Latency may be of two types, episomal and integrated. In the episomal state, both host and viral genes are required for replication of the agent.[20,21,24] The classic example of viral latency is that of varicella zoster. After an initial infection presenting as chicken pox, the viral genome is maintained in the sensory ganglia.[25,26] Reactivation of the latent viral infection produces herpes zoster along the cutaneous dermatomes, a condition also know as *shingles*. Reactivation involves replication of virus in the skin and peripheral mucus membranes to which the viral DNA has been transported from neural tissue. The neurons may continue to function as a permanent reservoir for the latent virus. A variety of agonists can trigger the reactivation from the latent to the active state. These include fever, trauma, ultraviolet light, and immunosuppression.[27]

Alternatively, the agent may be incorporated into the host genome. In some cases, such as adeno-associated virus, the viral genome is incorporated into a specific site.[28] In other cases, the site of integration is random. Hepatitis B virus, a small DNA-containing virus, integrates randomly into the genome.[29] Retroviral genomes are first reverse transcribed into a DNA intermediate which is then transported into the nucleus and incorporated into the host genome at sites of actively replicating DNA.[11,30] The viral genomes are flanked by long-terminal repeats that serve as sites of integration into the host genome, promoting the transcription of viral RNA. If the viral genome is not transcribed, the viral proteins are not translated and infectious viral particles are not generated. If the viral genome is transcribed, it may undergo another cycle of reverse transcription and integration into a new site, a process that is known as transposition.[31]

Viral latency may have phenotypic effects on the infected cells. The viral genome may express genes that affect the expression of host genes (*trans* effect).[32–35] Alternatively, the integrated viral genome may affect the expression of adjacent genes. When resting B cells are infected with Epstein-Barr virus (EBV) in the absence of cytotoxic T cells, lymphoblastoid cell lines are generated that are capable of growing permanently in culture. Each cell carries multiple copies of the viral genome and constitutively expresses the latent proteins, six nuclear antigens and three membrane proteins. Expression of the EBNA-1 nuclear antigen is associated with replication and maintenance of the EBV genome in the episomal state.[36] Expression of EBNA-2, EBNA-3c, and LMP1 cause high level expression of B-cell activation markers and cellular adhesion molecules; thus, the EBV-induced immortalization of B cells may function through the same cellular pathways that drive physiological B-cell proliferation.[37]

Transmission. Exogenous genetic agents are transmitted from one person to another in the presence or absence of direct contact. Viral aerosols and viral-bearing fomites may lead to uptake by the respiratory or gastrointestinal tracts. Entry via skin or direct inoculation into the bloodstream can occur through insect bites. Some viruses are transmitted only by direct exchange of body fluids.

When viruses are transmitted within a family they can mimic genetic inheritance. The pattern of transmission can be either horizontal, affecting multiple members of the same generation within a pedigree, or vertical, from parents to children (or vice versa). Vertical transmission occurs across the placenta (for HIV1)[38] or in the birth canal (for hepatitis) or both (for HSV).[39,40] Transmission can also occur via lactation.[41,42] In this way, viral transmission can demonstrate a parent-of-origin effect.

The severity and symptoms of disease can be variable between parents and children. Herpes and adenovirus infections can produce life-threatening illnesses in newborn infants.[43,44] In the absence of immunocompromise, disseminated herpes and cytomegalovirus (CMV) pneumonia are rare in older individuals.[45,46] By contrast, measles, mumps, and varicella produce more severe symptoms in adults than in children.[47] Congenital infection with agents such as cytomegalovirus and rubella can produce growth retardation, cerebral calcification, blindness, and deafness, symptoms that are never observed with postnatally acquired infections.[48,49] Congenital infections with these agents mimics genetic anticipation.

Prions. Several human neurodegenerative disorders, including Creutzfeld-Jakob disease (CJD),[50,51] Gerstmann-Straussler-Scheinker disease (GSS),[52] familial fatal insomnia (FFI), and kuru,[53] are slowly progressive. GSS and FFI are inherited as autosomal dominant conditions, whereas kuru is acquired as the result of infection from oral consumption or injection of human brain products.[54-56] CJD may be either inherited or acquired.[57-59] The presumed etiologic agent is PrP 27–30, a 30-kD protein that accumulates in amyloid-type plaques and results in a characteristic spongiform degeneration, gliosis, and neuronal loss in the absence of an inflammatory reaction.[13,60,61]

The PrP protein is encoded by a nuclear gene.[62,63] Mutations in the PrP gene are linked to the development of GSS, FFI, and CJD.[54,64-69] A novel form of protein, PrP^{CJD} or PrP^{Sc}, is found in the brain of most affected individuals.[13] The pathogenic form of the protein has a high ß-sheet content, is insoluble in detergents, and is relatively resistant to proteolysis.[70] This form differs from the normal cellular isoform, PrP^C, which is rich in α-helices and virtually devoid of ß-pleated sheet. The conversion of PrP^C to PrP^{CJD} appears to involve the unfolding of α-helices with refolding into ß-pleated sheets (Fig. 9.3).[71] For kuru and infectious CJD, the pathogenic form of the protein appears to be the only transmissible agent. No nucleic acid component has been identified. To emphasize the proteinaceous nature of the infectious agent, the term *prion* was developed.[70]

The animal model for prion diseases, scrapie, has provided additional evidence for the proteinaceous nature of the transmissible agent.[70] The titer of the infectious agent is proportional to the concentration of the PrP^{Sc} protein.[72,73]

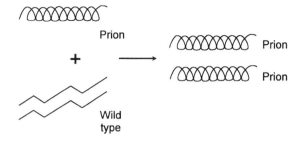

Figure 9.3. Prion particles induce conformational changes of wild-type isoforms of the same polypeptide.

The prion titer is reduced by denaturation or hydrolysis of PrP^{Sc} or by neutralization of with anti-PrP^{Sc} rabbit antisera.[74–76] Transgenic mice that were created with a GSS mutation in the mouse PrP gene (Pro101Leu) develop neurologic dysfunction, spongiform degeneration, and gliosis.[77] Transgenic mice that were created with the hamster PrP gene and then inoculated with the hamster prion developed amyloid plaques and scrapie infectivity that is characteristic of hamsters.[78,79] The PrP^{C} form can be converted to the PrP^{Sc} form in cell-free systems by incubation with exogenous PrP^{Sc}.[80] Taken together, these pieces of evidence suggest that the prion is a specific physical form of the PrP protein that causes the wild-type endogenous PrP protein to undergo a conformational shift into a similar pathogenic and infectious particle.[81] These particles represent a novel form of infectious agent transmission because they are not associated with their own nucleic acid. Moreover, these findings suggest that these neurodegenerative disorders may occur sporadically in the absence of infection if a PrP^{Sc} mutation occurs in the brain of an affected person.

MUTATIONAL EVENTS ASSOCIATED WITH HUMAN VIRUSES

Mutation associated with the agent. Viruses mutate from errors in replication or from recombination. The errors in replication may be point mutations or small insertions or deletions.[82] For retroviruses, the rate of mutation is 100- to 1,000-fold greater than it is in the nuclear genome.[83] Two factors contribute to the high rate of mutation. First, reverse transcriptase has a lower rate of fidelity than other cellular polymerases. Second, there is no enzymatic machinery to correct replication errors when these may occur.[47,84] High mutation rates occur for viruses that use RNA replicases, such a poliovirus, that do not copy their genomes through a DNA intermediate.[85]

Given the high rate of replication errors, variation at every base could arise in infected cells. In practice, viral genomes with specific sequence variants, termed *quasispecies,* are more prevalent (Fig. 9.4).[86,87] Selection may act to limit the degree of variability that occurs in viral genomes. The selection may be confined to viral sequences that have a replication advantage.[88]

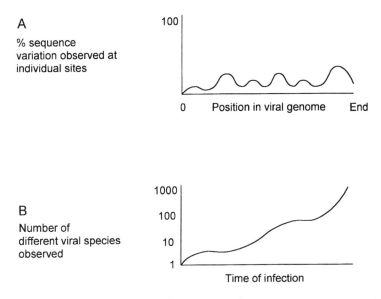

Figure 9.4. (A) Quasispecies are viral genomes with sequence variants around specific sites. (B) The number of quasispecies may increase over time.

Viruses also undergo recombination (Fig. 9.5). The recombination may be homologous, involving the same sites in other viral particles.[89] Homologous recombination leads to reshuffling of allelic genes between two viral genomes. Alternatively, the virus may undergo nonhomologous recombination with another virus or with the host genome.[90] Through the process of nonhomologous recombination, the virus may lose genes or acquire new genes.

Viruses that have acquired host genes as the result of nonhomologous recombinational events may infect other individuals. Although not yet demonstrated for humans, retroviruses have been shown to incorporate host DNA from mouse, chicken, and cat. The precursor RNA is processed into a mature mRNA molecule, which is then packaged and can infect other organisms.[30] This represents a novel means for transmitting genes among various members of a species.

A different means of recombination occurs with rotavirus, influenza virus, and other viruses that have segmented RNA genomes (Fig. 9.5). If a cell is infected with two genetically different rotavirus particles, different segments of the two viral genomes will be encapsidated, leading to a reshuffling of genes that is different from the parental types, a process called *reassortment.*[91]

Mutational events in the host. Following infection, there are two ways that a virus can alter the host genome. First, the agent may integrate into the coding region of a gene, disrupting its function. The disruption of the factor VIII gene by insertion of the retroviral-like L1 element represents such an event in certain

A: Non-segmented genomes

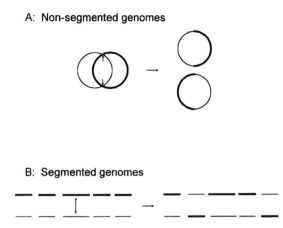

B: Segmented genomes

Figure 9.5. (A) Recombination between viral genomes may occur by exchange of genetic information between two different genomes. This may occur at homologous or nonhomologous sites. (B) Reassortment between segmented genomes occurs when different segments of two viral genomes are encapsidated, leading to a re-shuffling of genes that is different from the parental types.

cases of hemophilia A.[92] Second, the virus may integrate in the vicinity of a gene, altering its regulation. The promoter of the agent may cause the downstream gene to be expressed.[93] For example, the presence of long-terminal repeat sequences upstream of the 5' flanking regions of the three amylase genes is thought to contribute to their selective expression in salivary glands.[94] The high frequency of hepatitis B viral DNA integration in the genomes of infected hepatocytes is thought to contribute to the development of hepatocellular carcinoma.[29]

PHENOTYPIC EFFECTS IN THE HOST

Infection may be cytotoxic and lead to lysis and death of host cells in one of several ways (Fig. 9.6). First, the virus may inhibit the synthesis of host proteins and RNA by the cell. Different viruses use different mechanisms to inhibit synthesis of macromolecules. Poliovirus infection causes cleavage of the eIF-4F mRNA cap-binding complex.[95] Unlike host mRNAs, poliovirus RNA is not capped and therefore continues to be translated. Second, following infection the plasma membrane is damaged because cell protein and lipid synthesis ceases. The $Na+/K+$ gradient collapses, causing the $Na+$ concentration to rise and the $K+$ concentration to fall.[96] This may inhibit host protein translation. Other membrane transport processes may stop functioning. Third, lysosomal membranes may break down, causing the lysosomes to release their hydrolytic enzymes, causing further damage to host macromolecules.

A   Increase rate of cell-turnover

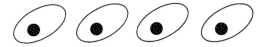

B   Immune/Inflammatory Response

C   Cell Death

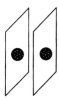

D   Cell Immortalization/Transformation

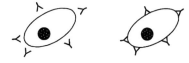

Figure 9.6. Phenotypic effects of viral infection. These include (A) increased rate of cell turnover, (B) immune/inflammatory response, (C) cell death, and (D) cell immortalization or transformation.

The toxicity of the virus may be augmented by the immune response that it evokes. Fixation of complement by antibodies or activation of cytotoxic T lymphocytes may lead to an inflammatory response with killing of uninfected cells, breakdown of capillary membrane barriers with interstitial edema, and loss of function. In the process of healing, the original cell types may be replaced with fibroblasts or other cells; hence, the function of the infected tissue may be altered permanently.[97] Even in the absence of an inflammatory response, the immune response may lead to a net loss of host cells. For example, long-term HIV infection leads to a net loss of CD4 T cells.[98]

The virus may alter the expression of host genes. Depending on the genes that are affected, this may have either a cytotoxic or a growth-promoting effect. Infection with almost all viruses leads to the expression of *interferons*, proteins that interfere with viral multiplication. Some animal retroviruses contain mutant copies of cell growth factors or their receptors that are called *proto-oncogenes.*[99] These retroviruses readily induce cancer in infected animals because their proto-oncogenes cause transformation in infected cells. Other viruses contain genes which when expressed will bind to anti-oncogene proteins that are present in the host cell. Binding of SV40 large T antigen or adenovirus E1 proteins to the anti-oncogenes p53 and Rb-1, respectively, lifts a block on cell division and proliferation.[100,101]

VIRAL INFECTION AND PUBLIC HEALTH

Viruses are one of nature's ways of introducing new genetic information into the host. As a result, they can be used to induce an immune response to specific antigens, including those directly encoded by the virus. Alternatively, they cause host cells to synthesize proteins that may be deficient or are not ordinarily made by the host.

Viruses as vaccines. One of the first indications of the infectious nature of viruses was the demonstration of their ability to induce an immune response in the host.[102] Edward Jenner observed that milkmaids who develop cowpox were immune to smallpox.[103] He found that he could protect susceptible individuals against smallpox by infecting them with cowpox *(vaccinia)*. Hence, the process of inducing an immune response by inoculating individuals with an infectious agent was called *vaccination*.[104] Louis Pasteur observed that an immune response could be induced by vaccination with the pathogen itself, rather than a related organism, and used this observation to develop vaccination procedures against cholera, anthrax, and rabies.[105] This procedure conferred some risk because the vaccinated individual could develop the disease prior to mounting an immune response.

To minimize the risks of vaccination, three different types of antiviral vaccines have been developed. The agents for these vaccines include inactivated virus, active but attenuated virus, and viral protein subunits.[106] Inactivated virus vaccines have lost infectivity with minimal loss of antigenicity. The best reagent for inactivating viral nucleic acids without loss of antigenicity is formaldehyde. By reacting with the free amino groups of guanine, adenine, and cytosine, formaldehyde destroys infectivity of viruses with single-stranded nucleic acids. Currently, this is the method that is used to prepare the influenza vaccine.[107]

The second type contains an active but attenuated virus. These attenuated strains replicate and induce an immune response in the host without causing disease.[108] The attenuated vaccines are effective at low doses because the virus can multiply in the host and the viral progeny act as the antigens. Prior to the availability of recombinant DNA technology, attenuated viruses were obtained by repeated passage of human pathogens in other host species and selection for variants with reduced virulence. Now that the genetics of human viruses are understood in considerable detail, human viruses have been attenuated by deleting or mutating viral genes.[109,110]

The advent of recombinant DNA technology has also led to the development of subunit vaccines. The development of these vaccines is based on the observation that some viral proteins may elicit a strong immune response. Viral proteins that have been synthesized in cultured cells, may then be purified for use as vaccines. Alternatively, the genes encoding these subunits have been cloned into nonvirulent vectors, such as attenuated vaccinia. The vaccinia has been attenuated by inactivation of the thymidine kinase and growth factor genes. When the recombinant vaccinia infects a host, the viral subunit gene is expressed and elicits an immune response.[111,112]

Viruses as agents of gene therapy. Gene therapy is the process of expressing foreign genes in humans to ameliorate a disease state.[113] Gene therapy is being used to replace gene products whose deficiencies are associated with genetic diseases, such as adenosine deaminase to treat the severe combined immunodeficiency that is associated with deficiency of that enzyme and LDL receptors to treat familial hypercholesterolemia. Another use is to express gene products that are novel to a given cell type. One such novel function is the development of tumor-infiltrating lymphocytes that express toxins. Tumor-infiltrating lymphocytes target human cancer cells. By engineering these cells to release toxins, such as interleukins or cholera toxin, it is hoped that they will kill tumors that are refractory to conventional forms of therapy.[114]

As nature's agents for introducing new genetic information into cells. human viruses are natural candidates as vectors for gene therapy.[4,115] The viral vector can have either a narrow or broad host range. For example, hepatitis B infects only hepatocytes, whereas human adenoviruses and retroviruses infect a broad range of cells.[116–118] The virus may be debilitated to prevent virulence. The expression of the gene in question may be controlled by inclusion of appropriate regulatory elements. The efficiency of infection in culture may be high. Furthermore, the virus may be integrated into the host genome for more stable transmission.

Gene therapy is predicated on the hypothesis that once incorporated the genetic information is stably transmitted by somatic cells. This hypothesis may be erroneous, at least given the current state of knowledge about stable genetic transmission. Replication errors, mitotic instability, and selection may all contribute to defy stable gene transmission.

The use of viral vectors may present other disadvantages. Some vectors cannot transmit large inserts. For example, adeno-associated virus will transmit inserts only of 8 kb or less.[117] Oniy a small proportion of the total number of cells in a tissue may be transformed. In the absence of positive selection, this may be insufficient to cause a therapeutic response. The host may mount an immune response against the viral antigens, resulting in destruction of infected cells. Alternatively, the virus may integrate into the host genome, resulting in cell death or cellular transformation. Successful strategies will require overcoming all of these barriers.

REFERENCES

1. Berns KI. Parvovirus replication. Microbiol Rev 54:316–329, 1990.
2. Caspar DLD, Klug A. Physical principles in the construction of regular viruses. Cold Spring Harb Symp Quant Biol 27:1–24, 1962.
3. Anderson MJ, Pattison JR. The human parvovirus. Arch Virol 82:137–148, 1982.
4. Howard CR. The biology of hepadnaviruses. J Gen Virol 67:1215–1235, 1986.
5. Howley PM, Broker TR. Papillomaviruses: Molecular and Clinical Aspects. New York: Alan R Liss, 1985.
6. Marion PL, Robinson WS. Hepadnaviruses: hepatitis B and related viruses. Curr Top Microbiol Immunol 105:99–121, 1983.
7. McGeoch DJ. The genomes of human herpesviruses: contents, relationships and evolution. Annu Rev Microbiol 43:235–265, 1989.
8. Nermut MV. The architecture of adenoviruses: recent views and problems. Arch Virol 64:175–196, 1980.
9. Fingeroth JD, Clabby ML, Strominger JD. Characterization of a T-lymphocyte Epstien-Barr virus/C3d receptor (CD21). J Virol 62:1442–1447, 1988.
10. Dalgleish AG, Beverley PC, Clapham PR, Crawford DH, Greaves MF, Weiss RA. The CD4 (T4) antigen is an essential component of the receptor for the AIDS retrovirus. Nature 312:763–767, 1984.
11. Weber T, Hunsmann G, Stevens W, Fleming AF. Human retroviruses. Baillieres Clin Haematol 5:273–314, 1992.
12. Brunk C. Formation of dimers in ultraviolet-irradiated DNA. Basic Life Sci 5A:61–65, 1975.
13. Prusiner SB. Novel proteinaceous particles cause scrapie. Science 216:136–144, 1982.
14. Alper T. Scrapie agent unlike viruses in size and susceptibility to inactivation by ionizing or ultraviolet radiation. Nature 317:750, 1985.
15. Pearse BMF. Clathrin and coated vesicles. EMBO J 6:2507–2512, 1987.
16. Marsh M, Helenius A. Virus entry into animal cells. Adv Virus Res 37:107–151, 1989.
17. Anonymous. Virus structure and assembly. Boston: Jones and Bartlett, 1985.
18. Stephens EB, Compans RW. Assembly of animal viruses at cellular membranes. Annu Rev Microbiol 42:489–516, 1988.
19. Iwasaki Y, Ohtani S, Clark HF. Maturation of rabies virus by budding from neuronal cell membranes in suckling mouse brain. J Virol 15:1020–1023, 1975.
20. Croen KD, Straus SE. Varicella-zoster virus latency. Annu Rev Microbiol 45:265–282, 1991.
21. Ho DY. Herpes simplex virus latency: molecular aspects. Prog Med Virol 39:76–115, 1992.
22. Baichwal VR, Sugden B. Latency comes of age for herpesviruses. Cell 52:787–789, 1988.
23. Roizman B, Sears AE. An inquiry into the mechanisms of herpes simplex virus latency. Annu Rev Microbiol 41:543–571, 1987.
24. Meier JL, Straus SE. Comparative biology of latent varicella-zoster and herpes simplex virus infections. J Infect Dis 166:S13-S23, 1992.
25. Stevens JG, Cook ML. Latent herpes simplex virus in sensory ganglia. Science 173:843–845, 1971.
26. Warren WG, Brown SM, Wroblewska Z, Gilden D, Koproski H, Subak-Sharpe J.

Isolation of latent herpes simplex virus from the superior cervical and vagus ganglions of human beings. N Engl J Med 298:1068–1070, 1978.

27. Blyth WA, Hill TJ, Field HJ, Harbour DA. Reactivation of herpes simplex virus infection by ultraviolet light and possible involvement of prostaglandins. J Gen Virol 33:547–550, 1976.

28. Kotin RM, Sinascalco M, Samulski RJ, Zhu X, Hunter L, Laughlin CA, et al. Site-specific integration by adeno-associated virus. Proc Natl Acad Sci USA 87:2211–2215, 1990.

29. Shafritz DA, Shouval D, Sherman HI, Hadziyannis SJ, Kew MC. Integration of hepatitis B virus DNA into the genome of liver cells of chronic liver disease and hepatocellular carcinoma. Studies in percutaneous liver biopsies and post-mortem tissue specimens. N Engl J Med 305:1067–1073, 1981.

30. Varmus H. Retroviruses. Science 240:1427–1435, 1989.

31. Boeke JD, Corces VG. Transcription and reverse transcription of retrotransposons. Annu Rev Microbiol 43:403–434, 1989.

32. Klein G. Viral latency and transformation: the strategy of Epstein-Barr virus. Cell 57:5–8, 1989.

33. Block TM, Spivack JG, Steiner I. A herpes simplex virus type I latency-associated transcript mutant reactivates with normal kinetics from latent infection. J Virol 64:3417–3426, 1990.

34. Sample J, Kieff E. Transcription of the Epstein-Barr virus genome during latency in growth-transformed lymphocytes. J Virol 64:1667–1674, 1990.

35. Stevens JG, Wagner EK, Devi-Rao GB, Cook ML, Feldman LT. RNA complementary to a herpes alpha gene mRNA is prominent in latently infected neurons. Science 235:1056–1059, 1987.

36. Lupton S, Levine AJ. Mapping genetic elements of Epstein-Barr virus that facilitate extrachromosomal persistence of Epstein-Barr virus-derived plasmids in human cells. Mol Cell Biol 5:2533–2542, 1985.

37. Wang F, Gregory C, Sample C, Rowe M, Liebowitz D, Murray R, et al. Epstein-Barr virus latent membrane protein (LMP1) and nuclear proteins 2 and 3c are effectors of phenotypic changes in B lymphocytes: EBNA-2 and LMP1 cooperatively induce CD23. J Virol 64:2309–2318, 1990.

38. Valente P, Main EK. Role of the placenta in perinatal transmission of HIV. Obstet Gynecol Clin North Am 17:607–617, 1990.

39. Prober CG, Sullender WM, Yasukawa LL, Au DS, Yeager AS, Arvin AM. Low risk of herpes simplex virus infections in neonates exposed to the virus at the time of vaginal delivery to mothers with recurrent genital herpes simplex virus infections. N Engl J Med 316:240–244, 1997.

40. Hutto C, Arvin A, Jacobs R, Steele R, Stagno S, Lyrene R, et al. Intrauterine herpes simplex virus infections. J Pediatr 110:97–101, 1987.

41. Lerondelle C, Greenland T, Jane M, Mornex JF. Infection of lactating goats by mammary instillation of cell-born caprine arthritis-encephalitis virus. J Dairy Sci 78:850–855, 1995.

42. Hainut P, Vaira D, Francois C, Calberg-Bacq CM, Osterrieth PM. Natural infection of Swiss mice with mouse mammary tumor virus (MMTV): viral expression in milk and transmission of infection. Arch Virol 83:195–206, 1985.

43. Hendersen JL, Weiner CP. Congenital infection. Curr Opin Obstet Gynecol 7:130–134, 1995.

44. Stamos JK, Rowley AH. Timely diagnosis of congenital infections. Pediatr Clin North Am 41:1017–1033, 1994.

45. Rubin RH, Tolkoff-Rubin NE. Opportunistic infections in renal allograft recipients. Transplant Proc 20:12–18, 1988.

46. Jules-Elysee K, Stover DE, Yahalom J, White DA, Gulati SC. Pulmonary complications in lymphoma patients treated with high-dose therapy autologous bone marrow transplantation. Am Rev Resp Dis 146:485–491, 1992.

47. Roberts JD, Bebenek K, Kunkel TA. The accuracy of reverse transcriptase from HIV-1. Science 242:1171–1173, 1988.

48. Dudgeon JA. Congenital rubella. J Pediatr 87:1078–1086, 1975.

49. Hanshaw JB, Schultx FW, Melish MM, Dudgeon JA. Congenital cytomegalovirus infections. Ciba Found Symp 10:23–43, 1972.

50. Creutzfeldt HG. Uber eine eignartige herdforminge Erkrankung des Zentrainervensystems. Z Gesante Neuro Psychiatr 57:1–18, 1920.

51. Jakob A. Uber eine der multiplen Sklerose klinisch nahestehende Erkrankung des Zentrainervensystems (sapstiche Pseudosklerose) mit bernerkenswerten anatomischern Belunde: Mittelung eines vierten Falles. Med Klin 17:372–376, 1921.

52. Gerstmann J, Straussler E, Scheinker I. Uber eine eigeartige heredtar-familare erkrankung des zentrainevensystem zugleich ein betrag zur frage des vorzeltigen lokalen alterns. Z Neurol 154:736–752, 1936.

53. Gajdusek C, Gibbs CJ, Alpers M. Slow-acting virus implicated in kuru. JAMA 199:34, 1967.

54. Collinge J, Harding AE, Owen F, Poulter M, Lofthouse R, Boughey AM, et al. Diagnosis of Gerstmann-Straussler syndrome in familial dementia with prion protein gene analysis. Lancet 2:15–17, 1989.

55. Gajdusek DC, Gibbs CJ, Jr., Alpers M. Experimental transmission of a kuru-like syndrome to chimpanzees. Nature 209:794–796, 1966.

56. Prusiner SB, McKinley MP, Groth DF, Bowman KA, Mock NI, Cochran SP, et al. Scrapie agent contains a hydrophobic protein. Proc Natl Acad Sci USA 78:6675–6679, 1981.

57. Gajdusek DC, Gibbs CJ, Jr., Rogers NG, Basnight M, Hooks J. Persistence of viruses of kuru and Creutzfeldt-Jakob disease in tissue cultures of brain cells. Nature 235:104–105, 1972.

58. Haltia M, Kovanen J, Van Crevel H, Bots GT, Stefanko S. Familial Creutzfeldt-Jakob disease. J Neurol Sci 42:381–389, 1979.

59. Gajdusek DC, Gibbs CJ, Jr. Transmission of two subacute spongiform encephalopathies of man (kuru and Creutzfeldt-Jakob disease) to new world monkeys. Nature 230:588–591, 1971.

60. Bockman JM, Kingsbury DT, McKinley MP, Bendheim PE, Prusiner SB. Creutzfeldt-Jakob disease prion proteins in human brains. N Engl J Med 312:73–78, 1985.

61. Wisniewski HM, Morets RC, Lossinsky AS. Evidence of induction of localized amyloid deposits and neuritic plaques by an infectious agent. Ann Neurol 10:517–522, 1981.

62. Basler K, Oesch B, Scott M, Westaway D, Walchli M, Groth DF, et al. Cellular and scrapie PrP isoforms are encoded by the same chromosomal gene. Cell 46:417–428, 1986.

63. Puckett C, Concannon P, Casey C, Hood L. Genomic structure of the human prion protein gene. Am J Hum Genet 49:320–329, 1991.

64. Medori R, Tritschler HJ, LeBlanc A, Villare F, Manetto V, Chen HY, et al. Fatal familial insomnia: a prion disease with a mutation at codon 178 of the prion protein gene. N Engl J Med 326:444–449, 1992.

65. Hsiao K, Baker HF, Crow TJ, Poulter M, Owen F, Terwilliger JD, et al. Linkage of a prion protein missense variant to Gerstmann-Straussler syndrome. Nature 338:342–345, 1989.

66. Hsiao K, Dlouhy S, Farlow MR, Cass C, DaCosta M, Conneally PM, et al. Mutant prion protein in Gerstmann-Straussler-Scheinker syndrome with neurofibillary tangles. Nat Genet 1:68–71, 1992.

67. Heston LL, Lother DLW, Leventhal CM. Alzheimer's disease: a familial study. Arch Neurol 15:225–233, 1966.

68. Owen F, Poulter M, Lofthouse R, Collinge J, Crow TJ, Risby D, et al. Insertion in prion protein gene in familial Creutzfeldt-Jakob disease. Lancet 1:51–52, 1989.

69. Goldfarb LG, Petersen RB, Tabaton M, Brown P, LeBlanc AC, Montagna P, et al. Creutzfeldt-Jakob disease: disease phenotype determined by a DNA polymorphism. Science 258:806–808, 1992.

70. Prusiner SB, Groth DF, Bolton DC, Kent SB, Hood LE. Purification and structural studies of a major scrapie prion protein. Cell 38:127–134, 1984.

71. Gasset M, Baldwin MA, Fleterick RJ, Prusiner SB. Perturbation of the secondary structure of the scrapie prion protein under conditions associated with infectivity. Proc Natl Acad Sci USA 90:1–5, 1993.

72. Bolton DC, McKinley MP, Prusiner SB. Identification of a protein that purifies with the scrapie protein. Science 218:1309–1311, 1982.

73. Prusiner SB, Groth DF, Cochran SP, Masizrz FR, McKinley MP, Martinez HM. Molecular properties, partial purification, and assay by incubation period measurements of the hamster scrapie agent. Biochemistry 19:4883–4891, 1980.

74. Neary K, Caughey B, Ernst D, Race RE. Protease sensitivity and nuclease resistance of the scrapie agent propogated in vitro in neuroblastoma cells. J Virol 65:1031–1034, 1991.

75. McKinley MP, Masiarz FR, Prusiner SB. Reversible chemical modification of the scrapie agent. Science 214:1259–1261, 1981.

76. Gabizon R, McKinley MP. Immunaffinity purification and neutralization of scrapie prion infectivity. Proc Natl Acad Sci USA 85:6617–6621, 1988.

77. Hsiao KK, Scott M, Foster D, Groth DF, DeArmond SJ, Prusiner SB. Spontaneous neurodegeneration in mice with mutant prion protein. Science 250:1587–1590, 1990.

78. Scott M, Foster D, Mirenda C, Serban D, Coufal F, Walchli M, et al. Transgenic mice expressing hamster prion protein produce species-specific scrapie infectivity and amyloid plaques. Cell 59:847–857, 1989.

79. Prusiner SB, Scott M, Foster D, Pan KM, Groth D, Mirenda C, et al. Transgenic studies implicate interactions between PrP isoforms in scrapie prion protein replication. Cell 63:673–686, 1990.

80. Bessen RA, Kocisko DA, Raymond GJ, Nandan S, Lansbury PT, Caughey B. Non-genetic propagation of strain-specific properties of scrapie prion protein. Nature 375:698–700, 1995.

81. Weissman C. A 'unified theory' of prion propogation. Nature 352:679–682, 1991.

82. Parvin JD, Moscona A, Pan WT. Measurements of the mutation rates of animal viruses: influenza V virus and poliovirus type 1. J Virol 59:377–383, 1986.

83. Dougherty JP, Temin HM. Determination of rate of base-pair substitution and insertions in retrovirus replication. J Virol 62:2817–2822, 1988.

84. Preston RD, Ploesz BJ, Loeb LA. Fidelity of HIV-1 reverse transcriptase. Science 242:1168–1171, 1988.

85. Kuge S, Kawamura N, Nomoto A. Strong inclination toward transition mutation in nucleotide substitutions by poliovirus replicase. J Mol Biol 207:175–182, 1989.

86. Hahn BH, Shaw GM, Taylor ME, Redfield RR, Markham PD, Salahuddin SZ, et al. Genetic variation in HTLV-III/LAV over time in patients with AIDS or at risk for AIDS. Science 232:1548–1553, 1986.

87. Steinhauer DA, Holland JJ. Rapid evolution of RNA viruses. Annu Rev Microbiol 41:409–433, 1987.

88. Holland JJ, de la Torre JC, Clarke DK, Duarte E. Quantitation of relative fitness and gene adaptability of clonal populations of RNA viruses. J Virol 65:2960–2967, 1991.

89. Brown SM, Ritchie DA. Genetic studies with herpes simplex virus type I. Analysis of mixed plaque-forming virus and its bearing on genetic recombination. Virology 64:32–42, 1975.

90. Huang CC, Hammond C. Nucleotide sequence and topography of chicken c-fps. Genesis of a retroviral oncogene encoding a tyrosine-specific protein kinase. J Mol Biol 181:175–186, 1985.

91. Garbarg-Chenon A, Bricout F, Nicolas JC. Study of genetic reassortment between two human rotaviruses. Virology 139:358–365, 1984.

92. Kazazian HH, Jr., Wong C, Youssoufian H, Scott AF, Phillips DG, Antonarakis SE. Hemophilia A resulting from de novo insertion of L1 sequences represents a novel mechanism for mutation in man. Nature 332:164–166, 1988.

93. Hayward WS, Neel BG, Astrin SM. Activation of a cellular oncogenes by promoter insertion in ALV-induced lymphoid leukosis. Nature 290:475–480, 1981.

94. Ting CN, Rosenberg MP, Snow CM, Samuelson LC, Meisler MH. Endogenous retroviral sequences are required for tissue-specific expression of a human salivary amylase gene. Genes Dev 6:1457–1465, 1992.

95. Etchison D, Smith K. Variations in cap-binding complexes from uninfected and polio-virus infected HeLa cells. J Biol Chem 265:7492–7500, 1990.

96. Foster KA, Micklem KJ, Agnarsdottir G, Lancashire CL, Bogomolova NN, Boriskin YS, et al. Myxoviruses do not induce non-specific alterations in membrane permeability early on in infection. Arch Virol 77:139–153, 1983.

97. Lanzavecchia A. Is the T-cell receptor involved in T-cell killing? Nature 319:778–780, 1986.

98. Krohn KJ, Antonen J, Valle SL, Kazakevicius R, Saxinger C, Gallo RC, et al. Clinical and immunological findings in HTLV-III infection. Cancer Res 45(9 Suppl):4612s-4615s, 1985.

99. Bishop JM. Cellular onogenes and retroviruses. Annu Rev Biochem 52:301–354, 1983.

100. Reich NC, Levine AJ. Specific interaction of the SV40 T antigen-cellular p53 protein complex with SV40 DNA. Virology 117:286–290, 1982.

101. Moran E. Interaction of adenoviral proteins with pRB and p53. FASEB J 7:880–885, 1993.

102. Mechnikov II. The Founders of Modern Medicine: Pasteur, Koch, Lister. New York: Walden, 1939.

103. LeFanu WR. Edward Jenner. Proc R Soc Med 66:664–668, 1973.

104. Burke DS. Joseph-Alexandre Auzias-Turenne, Louis Pasteur, and early concepts of virulence, attenuation, and vaccination. Perspect Biol Med 39:171–186, 1996.

105. Porter JR. Louis Pasteur sesquicentennial (1822–1972). Science 178:1249–1254, 1972.

106. Brown F. New approaches in viral vaccine development. Scand J Infect Dis (Suppl) 76:39–46, 1990.

107. Gwaltney JM, DeSanctis AN, Metzgar DP, Hendley JO. Systemic reactions to influenza B vaccine. Am J Epidemiol 105:252–260, 1977.

108. Zygraich N. Criteria in the evaluation of live intranasal influenza virus vaccines. Dev Biol Stand 33:141–150, 1976.

109. Murphy BR, Prince GA, Collins PL, Van Wyke Coelingh K, Olmstead RA, Spriggs MK, et al. Current approaches to the development of vaccines effective against parainfluenza and respiratory syncytial virus. Virus Res 11:1–15, 1989.

110. Goldfarb LG, Haltia M, Brown P, Nieto A, Kovanen J, McCombie WR, et al. New mutation in scrapie amyloid precursor gene (at codon 178)in Finnish Creutzfeldt-Jakob disease kindred. Lancet 337:425, 1991.

111. Chambers TM, Kawaoka Y, Webster RG. Protection of chickens from lethal influenza infection by vaccinia-expressed hemaglutinin. Virology 167:414–421, 1988.

112. Esposito JJ, Knight JC, Shaddock JH. Succesful oral rabbies vaccination of racoons with racoon poxvirus recombinants expressing rabies virus glycoprotein. Virology 165:313–316, 1988.

113. Anderson WF. Human gene therapy. Science 256:808–813, 1991.

114. Rosenberg SA, Aebersold P, Cornetta K, et al. Gene transfer into humans: immunotherapy of patients with advanced melanoma, using tumor-infiltrating lymphocytes modified by retroviral gene transduction. N Engl J Med 323:570–578, 1990.

115. Lever AML. Vectors. Biochem Soc Trans 19:379–382, 1991.

116. Boris-Lawrie K, Temin HM. The retroviral vector. Ann NY Acad Sci 716:59–71, 1995.

117. Muzyczka N. Use of adeno-associated virus as a general transduction vector for mammalian cells. Curr Top Microbiol Immunol 158:97–129, 1992.

118. Jaffe HA, Daniel C, Longnecker G, Metzyer M, Setoyuchi Y, Rosenfeld MA, et al. Adenovirus mediated in vivo gene transfer and expression in normal rat liver. Nat Genet 1:372–378, 1992.

10

Human Variation: Determinism or Chance?

Over the past century, the study of human genetics has evolved into a multifaceted discipline with a variety of specialized tools. The application of these tools has demonstrated how the common features of human growth and development, biochemistry and physiology, are transmitted from one generation to the next. Despite the seeming commonality of human inheritance, our individuality in health, in disease, and in aging can be explained by our genetic makeup. This chapter will review the many different genetic processes that have been identified, their effects on phenotypic expression, and the possibilities for identifying other, currently unknown, genetic processes.

THE MECHANISMS OF HUMAN GENETICS

Mechanisms common to germ and somatic cells. Some genetic processes are shared by germ and somatic cells, whereas others operate in specific cell types. Mechanisms that operate in germ cells typically affect either gene transmission or gene expression (Table 10.1), whereas those that operate in somatic cells typically affect only expression (Table 10.2). Mechanisms may operate in an early embryonic cell and affect both somatic and germ cells.

Processes common to germ cells and somatic cells include (1) the replication of DNA in all actively dividing cells and the transmission of chromosomes to progeny cells, (2) mechanisms for repairing damage and chromosomal breaks induced by radiation and free radicals, (3) mechanisms for exchange between the two chromatids of a replicating chromosome (sister chromosome exchange) or between the two chromosomes in a pair (recombination), (4) mechanisms for replicating and transmitting mitochondrial genomes, (5) expression of a similar repertoire of housekeeping genes that encode proteins necessary for cell structure, metabolism, replication, and protein synthesis.

Specific genetic mechanisms. Some genetic mechanisms are confined either to germ or to somatic cells (Tables 10.1 and 10.2). Meiosis, the process that accounts for Mendel's laws, is unique to germ cells. Genomic imprinting is established in germ cells, although manifested only in somatic cells,[1] and telomere repair is confined mostly to germ cells.[2] Sex chromosome expression varies markedly between oocytes and spermatocytes. In primary oocytes, both X chromosomes are active.[3] By contrast, in late-stage spermatocytes both X and Y chromosomes are inactive.[4] In addition, the recombination of immunoglobulin and T-cell receptor genes is confined to specific types of somatic cells.[5]

Some of the processes that regulate gene expression are confined to somatic cells. Proteins that activate transcription of certain genes may be expressed only in one cell type. Regulatory mechanisms that operate on contiguous blocks of genes, such as X chromosome inactivation and genomic imprinting, appear to operate only from the time of embryonic development onward.[1,6] Modification of RNA by editing or preferential splicing of two exons may be confined to somatic cells of specific types.[6–8] Nonetheless, the identification of these many

Table 10.1. Genetic Mechanisms that Affect Germ Cells

Process	Recognition
Replication	Phenotypic continuity
	Sporadic case
	Gonadal mosaicism
	Anticipation
Meiosis	Segregation of loci
	Independent assortment of alleles
	Nondisjunction
	Aberrant segregation of derived
	chromosome(s)
Sex chromosome transmission	Sex determination
	Sex-linked phenotype
Recombination	Linkage
	Unequal recombination (sporadic case)
Genomic imprinting	Parent of origin transmission
Mitochondrial transmission	Maternal transmission
	Heteroplasmy (with variable expressivity)
X chromosome reactivation in oocytes	Demonstration of two active alleles?
	Gonadal dysgenesis or ovarian failure
X and Y inactivation in spermatids	Demonstration of no active locus
	?Oligo/azospermia

Table 10.2. Genetic mechanisms that affect somatic cells

Normal process	Recognition
Replication	Normal growth and development
	Somatic mosaicism
Mitosis	Normal growth and development
	Somatic mosaicism
	Uniparental disomy
	Loss of heterozygosity
Somatic recombination	Somatic mosaicism
Sister chromatid exchange	Uniparental disomy
	Loss of heterozygosity
X chromosome inactivation	Sex differences in X-linked phenotypes
Mitochondrial transmission	Heteroplasmy (with variable expressivity)
Viral infection	Somatic mosaicism

processes is not sufficient to explain all of the deviations from Mendel's rules. Some deviations may be accounted for by environmental effects and others may be accounted for by processes that are just starting to be characterized.

Environmental effects. Not all maternally transmitted effects are mediated by genomic imprinting, the mitochondrial genome, or the X chromosome. The intrauterine environment may also demonstrate a maternal effect on fetal development. Mothers may transmit agents that are toxic to the fetus. Transmission of maternal anti-Rh antibodies across the placenta leads to destruction of the infant's red blood cells, causing *hydrops fetalis*.[9] Transmission of infectious agents such as rubella and cytomegalovirus results in congenital infection and disrupts fetal development.[10] Infants who are exposed to elevated concentrations of phenylalanine in utero as the result of maternal phenylketonuria (PKU) may have growth retardation, microcephaly, congenital heart disease, and developmental delay. These effects may be mitigated if the mother's diet is controlled during the pregnancy. In some instances, the factor that causes a maternal effect is unknown. The risk of unprovoked seizures is higher in the children of affected mothers than in those of affected fathers. This risk is independent of the use of anticonvulsants during pregnancy; thus the biological basis could be either genetic or environmental.[11]

NOVEL GENETIC PROCESSES

It is unlikely that all of the genetic processes have been identified. The genetic mechanisms for some conditions that demonstrate familial clustering, but whose transmission does not follow Mendelian ratios, are unknown. Some of these conditions, such as juvenile-onset diabetes mellitus and other autoimmune diseases, are termed *multifactorial* because multiple genes and environmental exposure are postulated to be involved.[12] as a result of identifying genetic markers that are aggregated in relatives who are affected with insulin-dependent diabetes mellitus (also called *juvenile-onset* or *type 1*), up to ten genes have been identified as risk factors for the development of this condition.[13] The HLA genes are known to play a role in the immune responses, but the genes associated with other linked markers have not been identified yet; thus, the genetic cascade that operates to produce disease has not been determined. Analysis of the transmission of these markers from parents to offspring and their partitioning among somatic tissues may provide insight into the genetic processes involved.

Segregation distortion and meiotic drive. Some conditions show a parental origin effect. Although these observations have been termed *genomic imprinting,* other mechanisms may be involved. The preferential transmission of one of the two parental alleles is called *segregation distortion.* This may be the result of postzygotic selection in the embryo or of selection in the germ cells, in which case the phenomenon is termed *meiotic drive.* An early example of segregation distortion was observed for transferrin, an iron-binding protein. The maternal transferrin genotype that is inherited influences the paternal transferrin alleles that are found in the offspring. If the maternal and paternal transferrin alleles are incompatible, spontaneous abortion occurs.[14] Segregation distortion has also been observed for HLA alleles in dizygotic twins. The likelihood that dizygotic twins will share one or two HLA-DR alleles is close to 95%, that is, much higher than would be predicted by Mendel's rules.[15] Preferential transmission of the HLA-DR4 allele has been observed from diabetic fathers to their affected and unaffected children (72.1% versus 55.6% for children of affected mothers).[16] This phenomenon is thought to explain the higher incidence of insulin-dependent diabetes mellitus among the offspring of affected fathers than of affected mothers.[17]

Meiotic drive has been observed for several conditions associated with expanded trinucleotide repeats, including dentatorubral-pallidoluysian atrophy (DRPLA), Marchado-Joseph disease (MJD), and myotonic dystrophy.[18,19] Although seemingly autosomal dominant conditions, the number of affected offspring was greater than the number of unaffected offspring. This distortion favoring mutant alleles was found for the offspring of affected males. For DRPLA this included 62% of offspring and for MJD 72%. For each of these conditions, the instability of the trinucleotide repeat is more common in male, rather than female, germ cells, suggesting the possibility of a common mechanism between the genetic instability and the meiotic drive. By contrast, segregation distortion has been disproven for cystic fibrosis, a condition that is not associated with expanded trinucleotide repeats.[20] Direct genetic analysis of sperm cells has demonstrated equal transmission of normal and mutant alleles among fathers who are carriers for cystic fibrosis.

Parental origin effects and somatic chromosomal stability. Parental origin effects have also been observed for sporadic osteogenic sarcomas and neuroblastomas. Preferential loss of the maternal RB1 allele has been observed in over 90% of sporadic osteogenic sarcomas.[21] Since these tumors were of late onset and not preceded by retinoblastomas, it is thought that they contained somatic rather than germline mutations in their paternal RB1 alleles. As a result, the preferential loss of maternal alleles could not be explained by differences in the rate of paternal germline mutations.

Amplification of a segment of genomic DNA containing the MYCN oncogene is a frequent finding in advanced-stage neuroblastoma. The presence of this amplification carries a poor prognosis. When the parental origin was examined, the amplification occurred preferentially for the paternal MYCN allele.[22] To date, no differences in expression have been observed for the maternal and paternal alleles of RB1 and MYCN. Thus, these genes do not appear to be imprinted. Rather, these events may represent differences in the structures of the maternally and paternally derived chromosomes, leading to differences in the rates of deletion or gene amplification.

Methods for proving a genetic mechanism. The identification of a new genetic mechanism should meet several criteria to confirm the role of the mechanism in the development of a specific phenotype. First, the process should demonstrate a nonrandom association with a given phenotype that can be rigorously tested using a statistical method, such as LOD scores (for linkage) or χ^2 analysis (for association). Second, the strength of the association should increase as the markers analyzed approach the gene(s) that causes the condition. Third, there should be a biological assay that demonstrates that the expression of a causative gene has been altered as the result of the genetic mechanism.

GENETIC DETERMINISM AND ITS LIMITS

The mechanisms of gene transmission and gene regulation are conservative. The genome provides the blueprint for de novo macromolecular synthesis and organelle assembly. Newly synthesized molecules are built onto a preexisting molecular template, leading to the development of progeny cells. In turn, the migration and assembly of cells that form organs are mediated by recognition processes that are genetically encoded. If all went according to plan, an individual's development could be accurately predicted at the time of conception and monozygotic twins would be truly identical. Any variation would be attributable only to differences in environmental exposures.

The view that the phenotype of the organism is completely laid out by its genetic constitution is known as *genetic determinism*. Although genetic processes operate in a predictable way, there are limits to their determinism. First, these processes may be error-prone. New mutations, somatic recombination, and chromosomal nondisjunction occur with measurable frequency in each person every day. Because the error rate exceeds the number of bases in a cell's genome, the progeny cells are unlikely to be identical to their parental cell types. The rate at which errors accumulate may be accelerated by mutant proofreading genes whose products perform their functions imperfectly and thus act as mutator, rather than corrective, agents.

Second, some genetic processes are variable or stochastic in their occurrence. A priori, the choice of X chromosome to inactivate or nuclear or mitochondrial genome to transmit may be completely subject to chance. As a result, the genetic constitution of the progeny cells cannot be predicted with certainty. The distribution of cells within a tissue may be completely random or may have gone through selection or genetic drift. As a result, certain types of genetic constitutions may be overrepresented among an individual's population of cells.

Third, genetic processes may be modified by environmental exposures. Some agents, such as viruses or ionizing radiation, may have a direct mutagenic on genes. The net effect of such exposures is to increase the rate at which genetic errors occur and are propagated. Other environmental agents may interact with gene products to alter transcription, enzyme activity, signal transduction, or protein conformation. If applied for only a short time, such exposures may be reversible. If applied for longer periods of time, such exposure may produce irreversible effects.

Somatic genetic variation occurs in a person over the course of his or her lifetime. If the whole person were sampled, small populations of cells would be found that contained mutations for one or more genes. Chromosomal constitution and levels of gene expression would vary from cell to cell. Over time, the relative proportions of cells of a given genotype would vary. In addition, cells with new genotypes would appear. Some cells would gain new functions. Other cells would lose their replication potential or would die. When the accumulated genetic effects resulted in loss of homeostasis, illness and ultimately death occur.

Prediction of phenotype. Human geneticists seek to predict an individual's phenotype based on analysis of his or her genotype. If genetic processes operated in a completely deterministic way, it would be possible to predict outcomes based on knowledge of the 100,000–200,000 alleles in each individual. However, the power of prediction based on knowledge of phenotype is limited in two ways. The first is biologic. The genome is dynamic and the genetic constitution of a given cell may change over time. In addition, genetic processes are stochastic, so that even if the makeup of the genome did not change over time, the exact genetic constitution of somatic cells could not be predicted with accuracy.

The second limitation is observer-related. Our current understanding of the interactions of the various alleles of different genes is limited. A single gene may exert a profound effect in some people but may have its effects diluted by the genetic constitutions of other people. Certain genes may modify or negate the expression of other genes. For humans, analysis of multigene or epistatic interactions is still in its infancy. Currently, most predictions of phenotype based on genotype must be expressed in terms of probabilities, reflecting the residual uncertainty. A better understanding of genetic modifiers will lead to more precise predictions of phenotype based on genotype.

DEVELOPMENT OF A NEW CONCEPTUAL FRAMEWORK

This book has presented a conceptual framework for human genetics, emphasizing those phenomena that are exceptions to Mendel's rules. This framework is based on genetic mechanisms that have been identified up to this point in time. This framework will continue to evolve as new discoveries are made.

Identification of all human genes. It is anticipated that within a few years virtually all of the genes in the human genome will be identified. This will be accomplished by sequencing clones from human cDNA libraries. In turn, these will provide the framework for sequencing the entire human genome.

Identification of gene functions. As these genes are identified, so, too, will their functions. Some functions will be predicted based on sequence homologies. Others will be identified from their association with phenotypes in humans. The functions of other, unknown, genes will be determined by testing for effects in transgenic animals. Some will prove to be completely novel and will result in previously unidentified phenotypes. Others will result in phenotypes for which counterparts have been identified in humans.

During the next several years, it is likely that the factors that mediate genomic imprinting, X chromosome inactivation, and other modifiers of gene expression will be identified. This will provide new insights into whether processes that we now consider to be homogeneous in fact are. In addition, greater emphasis will be placed on studying germ cell development. This will yield insight into whether as-yet-unidentified processes exist that influence the transmission or subsequent expression of genes. The identification of genes and their functions and the processes that mediate their transmission and expression will provide the basis for understanding how genes interact with one another and may act as modifiers. In turn, this will make the prediction of phenotype, based on genotype, more precise.

The identification of so many genetic processes and the recognition that they occur on a daily basis in each of us will change how we think about human genetics. We all face risks from inheriting or acquiring deleterious alleles. Our successes in meeting the challenges of our environment are in part determined by the time in our life cycle during which they occur. Our successes are also determined by avoidance of agents that are toxic to our genomes, or when possible, by immunization against agents that we cannot avoid.

Our genes provide us with the potential to maximize our accomplishments and our survival. For the most part, we learn about our biological potential by testing ourselves as we take on the challenges of our lives. In the future, we may be able to predict the keys to our accomplishments and survival by knowledge of our genotypes.

REFERENCES

1. Howlett SK. Genomic imprinting and nuclear totipotency during embryonic development. Int Rev Cytol 127:175–192, 1991.
2. Sharma HW, Sokolski JA, Perez JR, Maltese JR, Sartorelli AC, Stein CA, et al. Differentiation of immortal cells inhibits telomerase activity. Proc Natl Acad Sci USA 92:12343–12346, 1995.
3. Kratzer PG, Chapman VM. X chromosome reactivation in the oocytes of Mus caroli. Proc Natl Acad Sci USA 78:3093–3097, 1981.
4. Tres LL. Nucleolar RNA synthesis of meiotic prophase spermatocytes in the human testis. Chromosoma 53:141–151, 1975.
5. Mak TW. Molecular similarities and differences between immunoglobulin and T cell receptors. Behring Inst Mitt 87:1–9, 1990.
6. Gartler SM, Dyer KA, Goldman MA. Mammalian X chromosome inactivation. Mol Genet Med 2:121–160, 1992.
7. Andreadis A, Gallego ME, Nadal-Ginard B. Generation of protein isoform diversity by alternative splicing: mechanistic and biological implications. Annu Rev Cell Biol 3:207–242, 1987.
8. Melcher T, Maas S, Herb A, Sprengel R, Seeburg PH, Higuchi M. A mammalian RNA editing enzyme. Nature 379:460–464, 1996.
9. Weiner AS. Genetic theory of the Rh blood groups. Proc Soc Exp Biol Med 54:316–319, 1943.
10. Hendersen JL, Weiner CP. Congential infection. Curr Opin Obstet Gynecol 7:130–134, 1995.
11. Ottman R, Annegers JF, Hauser WA, Kurland LT. Higher risk of seizures in offspring of mothers than of fathers with epilepsy. Am J Hum Genet 43:257–264, 1988.
12. Adams DD, Adams YJ, Knight JG, McCall J, White P, Horrocks R, et al. A solution to the genetic and environmental puzzles of insulin-dependent diabetes mellitus. Lancet 1:420–424, 1984.
13. Cordell HJ, Todd JA. Multifactorial inheritance in type I diabetes. Trends Genet 11:499–504, 1995.
14. Weitkamp LR, Schacter BZ. Transferrin and HLA: spontaneous abortion, neural tube defects, and natural selection. N Engl J Med 313 (15):925–932, 1985.
15. Jawaheer D, MacGregor AJ, Gregersen PK, Silman AJ, Ollier WER. Unexpected HLA haplotype sharing in dizygotic twin pairs discordant for rheumatoid arthritis. J Immunol 1997.
16. Vadheim CM, Rotter JI, Maclaren NK, Riley WJ, Anderson CE. Preferential transmission of diabetic alleles within the HLA gene complex. N Engl J Med 315 (21):1314–1317, 1986.
17. Warram JH, Krolewski AS, Gottlieb MS, Kahn CR. Differences in risk of insulin-dependent diabetes in offspring of diabetic mothers and diabetic fathers. N Engl J Med 311:149–151, 1984.
18. Ikeuchi T, Igarashi S, Takiyama Y, Onodera O, Oyake M, Takano H. Non-Mendelian transmission in dentatorubral-pallidolusian atrophy and Marchado-Joseph disease:

the mutant allele is preferentially transmitted in male meiosis. Am J Hum Genet 58:730–733, 1996.

19. Carey N, Johnson K, Nokelainen P, Peltonen L, Savontaus ML, Juvonen V, et al. Meiotic drive at the myotonic dystrophy locus? Nat Genet 6:117–118, 1994.

20. European Working Group on Cystic Fibrosis Genetics. No evidence for segregation distortion of cystic fibrosis alleles among sibs of cystic fibrosis patients. Eur J Hum Genet 3:324–325, 1995.

21. Toguchida J, Ishizaki K, Sasaki MS, Nakamura Y, Ikenaga M, Kato M, et al. Preferential mutation of paternally derived RB gene as the initial event in sporadic osteosarcoma. Nature 338:156–158, 1989.

22. Cheng JM, Hiemstra JL, Schneider SS, Naumova A, Cheung N-KV, Cohn SL. Preferential amplification of the paternal allele of the N-myc gene in human neuroblastomas. Nat Genet 4:191–193, 1993.

Index